EXTREME
TRANSFORMATION

CHRIS POWELL
AND
HEIDI POWELL

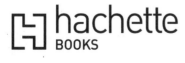 hachette
BOOKS

NEW YORK   BOSTON

Heidi's Dedication:

To my best friend. If people only knew the highs and lows we have endured together. Through it all, you've shown me generous acts of love and kindness even when I feel like I least deserved it. You make me want to be the best version of myself possible. Sometimes I have to pinch myself to make sure I'm really living this life as your other half. You are most definitely my better half. You've taught me more than you will ever know by your shining example. I can't wait to grow old with you, Chris.

Chris's Dedication:

To my best friend, Heidi. My world changed forever the day we met. You have taught me the most valuable lessons in this life. Our ride has certainly been a wild one. But when it is all said and done here, I cannot wait to look into your eyes, hand in hand, and know in our hearts that we did it all.

CONTENTS

PART FIVE
EXTREME CYCLE RECIPES

APPENDICES

INTRODUCTION

CREED OF THE PHOENIX

I found myself
Lost in the depths
Of darkness and despair,
Blinded by confusion
That was dwelling everywhere.

No matter how many times I tried
I couldn't find my way.
But when I opened up my eyes
A whole new life awaited.

Through hope and heart and promises,
Integrity and dignity,
My life is now my masterpiece.
I control my destiny.

I am a Phoenix now
From ash I rise above
As I climb, step-by-step
The path to true self love.

The Phoenix is a mythical bird that, near the end of its lifetime, crashes into the earth in a ball of flames—and then reincarnates itself to begin life anew.

It has been six years since we started our show *Extreme Weight Loss*—six seasons, over 70 incredible transformations on camera, and millions of lives changed in more than 140 countries! So much has happened in that short span of time—our family has expanded, our passion for helping others continues to grow, and our insight into how people can effectively lose weight and get in shape has deepened. But one of the biggest transformations of all is how we finally understand the necessary steps to keeping it off forever.

Since Heidi became even more visible on the show, the response has been overwhelming. People want more of her—on the show and via her blog, HeidiPowell.net. But what many don't realize is that Heidi and I have worked side by side from day one, helping our people change their lives for the better. As Heidi's role on the show has increased, I've been super excited—but not a bit surprised—to see how our viewers have responded to her amazing spirit, energy, and wisdom. They seem to relate to her emotionally charged, dig-in approach; instead of backing off when things get tough, Heidi helps them through some of the tough inner parts of their struggle to lose weight and hold steady to their transformation journey . . . and ultimately their lifelong dreams.

It turns out that my strengths as head cheerleader and chief educator dovetail nicely with Heidi's more emotional approach. Don't get me wrong: We are both tough, but in different ways, and we came to realize that the most successful of the people we work with need just that: cheerleader, educator, and counselor. They also have relied upon us as trusted friends—and that's what we want to be to you, friends you can depend on—to be honest with you, and to help guide you to your best life.

Together, we have always felt like a formidable team, but now with so many people responding to us as a couple (and family), we realize that yes, two is better than one . . . and our differences support our approach. And that's what we want to give you in this third—our most comprehensive and complete—book: a combination of both our approaches through a 21-day lifestyle shift that will put you on course to change your body and your life, forever.

Since our last book, we have made some influential discoveries—influential on *us*! Taking in the experience of the hundreds of courageous women and men we have guided through the weight loss journey, we've learned *so* much more about the struggles, and how to overcome them for continued success. We have dug deep with our people over the years, and now deliver to you the fastest, most convenient, most balanced way to achieve profound weight loss. Over the years we have set out to identify the reasons why it is so difficult for many to not just lose the weight, but to continue losing weight over time, and ultimately maintain a lifestyle of success. Why? Why do we lose motivation? Why do we fall off of the wagon time and again? How can we finally lose the weight for good? These are the questions that we have obsessed over for years and have sought tirelessly to find the solutions.

The answer is simple: Most diets are just that—diets. They are simple plans to follow for weight loss. Some even come with an exercise component. But they don't provide the inner compass, the knowledge, and the realistic expectations of what the journey is *really* like, to make a diet into what it's meant to be—*a transformation*. Before, there was no real *guide* to transformation. And that's our promise to you: a complete road map that will lead to long-term success—once and for all.

Our guide to Extreme Transformation is a product of over 14 years of experience on a journey that we've taken with hundreds of people. Nearly every individual we have transformed is like family to us. We talk, we laugh, we cry, and we have totally open and authentic communication about their struggles and triumphs—and through this experience we have gleaned *so* much about the pitfalls and how to prevent them, during both the weight loss journey and maintenance.

The weight loss technique we use for Extreme Transformation is the most complete and powerful nutrition and exercise plan we have ever designed. It is based upon our insight into the people who not only lose the weight, but also keep it off. Within each of the 21 days is a fundamental lesson that we have discovered to have a lasting impact upon every single transformation achieved. This approach leads to true, lasting success—the kind we are all interested in. We give them the tools to not only maximize their weight loss but also *stay* active and fit. These tools and fundamental lessons make this possible and set them apart from the millions of yo-yo dieters out there. They continue to practice these simple 21 lessons every day.

We have analyzed exactly what makes these *most* successful people do so well on our program. You're about to meet many of them, hear their stories, and see their remarkable transformations in their before-and-after photos.

When you witness their journeys of success, you will be inspired and motivated to declare your own dream as well—because if *they* can do it, you can, too—whether you're trying to lose just 20 pounds, or well over 100.

If you, your client, your family member, or your loved one wants Extreme Transformation and wants to change life forever, this is your guide. We are ready to give full transparency to our whole approach, and give you real-life expectations of what is to come. Woven into these 21 days are rules, tips, tricks, and shortcuts that we will share with you—from tactics that can accelerate your weight loss, to shifting the way you think about yourself and about weight loss forever.

This same method that we use to take 50 to 200 pounds off our participants in less than a year is the *same* one we've effectively used for hundreds of other clients who want to lose just 10 to 15 pounds! Not only does it help them achieve their weight loss goals, but it also sets them up for lifelong success. Early on, we'll help you see and understand the hidden path of transformation, which usually coincides with a big "a-ha" moment, and once you "get it," you will never see life or the weight loss journey the same way again. Whether it's the final 20 pounds or more than 200 that you want to lose, just follow the program, apply the lessons, and the results will be phenomenal. Best of all, along the way we'll show you how to control the throttle, so you can drop weight at a slower, more comfortable pace, or accelerate to get to your goal in record time.

We applied the science behind behavior and habits, alongside our own personal experience, with our participants: what is necessary to break a bad habit and how we can lay down new, positive habits. We found what worked and didn't work in their real-life situations, and have filtered it down to the most effective, tangible steps toward lifelong change.

You may have heard that it takes 21 days to change a habit, and while many of us can change a habit in 21 days, recent research by such behavioral scientists as Ann M. Graybiel has shown that, for some of us, it can take longer. We're not telling you this to worry you but instead to educate you and give realistic expectations of the journey ahead. The good news is that we have planned around this. We have structured our nutrition and exercise method in 21-day phases so that you learn how to change the bad habits that led to your weight gain and replace them with new, empowering habits that help you lose weight and feel much better. You can repeat the 21-day phase until you've reached your goal weight and replaced those destructive habits with new routines to "anchor in" your new body and mind-set.

As you can see, this is *the* guide to total transformation. These are *all* of our secrets. This transformation you are about to embark upon will lead to a whole new you. It is a kind of change that is deep and life altering. It is not superficial. It is not just physical change; it is an emotional, mental, social, and even spiritual change. It's the kind of change that takes all of you—your thoughts and your feelings, your body and your brain. All of you.

Now, we aren't just going to sit here, telling everyone else to follow these 21 lessons. No, we actually practice and follow them ourselves. We are so passionate about this process because these steps have enriched and changed *our* lives! Yes. We live Extreme Transformation on a daily basis. So when we teach you the lessons of transformation, we are sharing with you not just as your coaches, but also as your equals—your teammates on this journey. These steps are lessons that we'll never master—but to live our best life, we must continually practice them! We're all in this together. While you are living Extreme Transformation, know that we, and hundreds of thousands of other people are, too!

We've also included tips—some from Heidi, and some from me. You'll know who's talking to you by these clever little icons that tag them:

When you follow the 21 days of the Extreme Carb Cycle (our nutrition plan) and Metabolic Missions (our exercise plan), you will see and feel your body change rapidly. But when you learn and apply the lessons within the 21 Days to Transformation, you will feel a whole new sense of control over your life and your destiny. Finally, after years of feeling lost, depressed, or frustrated, you will come to a place where you feel hopeful and optimistic. You will see your life and your future with clarity. You will wake up in the morning with enthusiasm. You will go through your day confident and self-assured. You will turn out the light at night feeling successful, satisfied, and in control.

The 21 Days to Transformation fall into three weeks, each week covering one of the three components to create your own Extreme Transformation. Your days begin with good ol' delicious nutrition and a workout challenge, followed by one transformation lesson and activity that creates a deeper understanding of who you are and how you can unlock your true potential.

Week One: Days 1–7 help you **Learn It**

Week Two: Days 8–14 help you **Love It**

Week Three: Days 15–21 help you **Live It** for the rest of your life!

This is our promise to you: We will show you how to lose weight, get fit, and discover a part of you that you never knew existed. You will feel confident and energetic—able to take on life's challenges with vigor. You will feel happier and more in control than ever before. You will love yourself. That's what Extreme Transformation can do for you.

Let the journey begin...

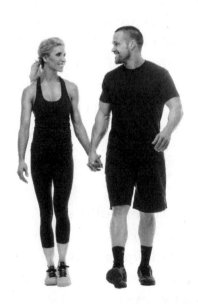

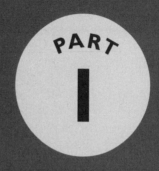

PART

I

The Method

Chapter One

WHY EXTREME TRANSFORMATION?

Our hit show *Extreme Weight Loss* has inspired millions of men and women around the world to change their lives for the better. In the show, we guide our courageous participants through a year-long journey of transformation. Although they lose hundreds of pounds in the process, the most rewarding part is what they gain: confidence, self-esteem, love, courage, and the know-how to control their bodies for the rest of their lives.

Our goal for this book is to share every component, every lesson, every aspect of transformation that will enable you to reach your weight loss goals and live enthusiastically—for the rest of your life. Though we've designed this 21-day guide around the exact method that we use with our participants, we have fine-tuned it so that whether you are here to lose those pesky 10 pounds that you put on and take off like a yo-yo, the last 20 pounds of post-baby weight, or 100 pounds or more, you can consider these 21 action-packed days your personal transformation boot camp—your guide to lifelong weight loss. We feel that this is the most effective method to date because it builds on our previous strategies and successes over the years, and includes new improvements that can deliver significant weight loss (as much as 1.5 percent of your body weight per week if you choose).

The 21-day plan is built upon a simple but powerful carb-cycle approach to eating, a once-a-day brief exercise *mission* that will stimulate your muscles and activate your body for weight loss, a fun activity of your choosing to accelerate your weight loss, and a simple yet powerful lesson and mental activity. This may sound routine, but let us assure you—the transformation journey you are about to embark upon is anything but!

We know that most diets can work—at least in the short term. Heck, a quick Internet search will find literally hundreds of plans that will most likely get you to take off weight if you follow them correctly. Unfortunately most diets don't take into account the necessary mental strategies, tactics, and know-how to control your weight for the rest of your life. So what happens? You lose weight in the short term, but then inevitably you go back to your old habits and patterns and gain it all back.

This is why Extreme Transformation is nothing like a diet. Instead, our no-nonsense approach to transformation contains within it our 21 simple but crucial lessons that clear the way for you to change your relationship with food and alter the habits that led to your weight gain to begin with. In these pages, we will lay out the entire journey for you—the good, the bad, and the ugly. We don't want to sugarcoat what lies ahead. Changing deeply engrained habits will get you out of your comfort zone and you will have moments—or days—of uneasiness and challenges. But we believe that if you face this inevitable discomfort head-on, you will find a sense of personal strength you never thought possible. So if you are ready to lose the weight forever, look no farther. But be prepared: There is some tough love ahead!

We realize that if you've picked up this book, you are already open to this process. You've taken an essential step toward a better life. But listen closely: True and lifelong transformation digs much deeper than diet and exercise. The process of losing excess pounds? That's the easy part. Really. And that's where we are going to start. We are going to show you the very simple, straightforward way to eat and exercise that will help you lose all the weight you want to lose. We'll show you how and why it works. We'll give you the exact method we use to help people lose up to hundreds of pounds in less than a year. You are going to be eating delicious foods (and we have included dozens of easy-to-prepare recipes for each day of the 21-day cycle) and discovering just how easy and rewarding the Metabolic Missions and Accelerators are.

As soon as you shift into this weight loss mode, you will begin to lose weight, feel lighter, and be more energetic! And that's just the beginning.

After one week, your body will begin to shed unwanted water weight and fat, and show signs of a more efficient metabolism. In two weeks you will see and feel a significant change in your body, and by the third week you will begin to feel more confident and clear about reaching your goals…and your life. You'll begin to see and believe that you really *can* do this.

We give you all that you need to do—a day-by-day road map that will get you to your weight loss goals (see chapter 2 for more details on how the carb cycle works). Each day offers five meals, a quick 5- to 20-minute Metabolic Mission, a weight loss Accelerator, and a fundamental lesson and mental activity to stoke your motivation and create a deeper understanding of yourself so that you can keep the weight off forever. All your meals—breakfast, lunch, snacks, and dinner—are laid out for you so you don't have to do any thinking! And we've also included some "Clean Cheat" snacks and meals for your reward days, too! Just follow the path!

These days are set up so that we can all go through the plan together. Day 1 through Day 4 we rev up our metabolism and burn fat with healthy carbs, Metabolic Missions, and Accelerators. Come Day 5, we all switch to low-carbs, turbocharging our weight loss for two days so we can all step on the scale the morning of Day 7 and see our amazing progress. If you want the same experience our participants go through on the show, this is it. In fact, as you are going through this *right now*, our participants and thousands of people around the world are, too!

Of course, if your work or living schedule doesn't match up with a Monday-through-Sunday schedule, no problem. You can start your Extreme Cycle on any day of the week—just choose what best fits with you. The 21-day cycle is flexible and adaptable to you, your goals, and your lifestyle.

But the beauty is that in just 21 days, you will begin a powerful and effective way to lose weight and get in shape. You will lose a number of pounds weekly and feel lighter, more fit, and more confident in just 21 days. You will maximize your metabolism so that your body can mobilize and oxidize fat effectively. You will also become more finely attuned to your body's response to food so that you feel satisfied, balanced, and no longer at the mercy of out-of-control cravings. And if you ever do experience a craving, we show you all of the tricks of the trade to curb it instantly, so that you always remain in control.

Our new exercise plan is part of this metabolic remake: These 15 Metabolic Missions will challenge you to explore your physical capabilities of running, jumping, pushing, crunching, and squatting so that you boost metabolism, and shape and develop lean muscle. You will begin to see an entirely new, more slender and cut silhouette. Just look at the dozens of before-and-after photos of our peeps in the pages ahead, and see what they created for themselves through Extreme Transformation! Best of all, you will repeat the 15 Metabolic Missions every three weeks, and when you perform them again you will perform more reps and more rounds than before. Every 21 days, you will see quantitative proof that you are getting fitter! These missions are designed to turn you into a badass.

Each Metabolic Mission is simple and easy to work into your daily routine. You will not have to carve out huge sections of time to fit in a complicated fitness program. You don't need any equipment. And you don't even need to go to a gym if you prefer exercising at home! You will be able to do a quick, effective workout in less than 15 to 20 minutes a day, five days a week. Accelerators are an added bonus that are included to boost your metabolism and burn even more fat. These longer-duration exercises (think cardio) are optional—but once you learn how they actually accelerate your weight loss, we won't need to convince you. Ultimately, they can lead to your record-breaking weight loss!

Eating and exercising are just the beginning of your transformation journey. In fact, they're the easy part. The secret ingredient to your life of transformation lies in the motivational lessons that accompany each of the 21 Days to Transformation.

HOW EXTREME TRANSFORMATION REALLY WORKS

We do things a little differently around here. Yes, you are going to follow the exact diet and exercise plan that we use for all of our remarkable transformations, but we have found that when you are able to "see" weight loss from a different perspective, you will focus on something totally different than the diet and exercise, and actually embrace this process with *enthusiasm*. Anybody can reluctantly follow a diet plan and lose weight…but think about what we're actually saying here: Imagine going through this weight loss journey and arriving into maintenance, without ever having to fixate on diet and exercise. That's right. Granted, we will teach you diet and exercise, but you're going to feel so good focusing on the true components of transformation, the weight loss just happens. We are going to show you how to radically shift your thinking to do just that, which is why your results will be so extraordinary!

In the process, you will identify different aspects of your life that have been holding you back, preventing you from achieving an extraordinary life. We understand how overwhelming and uncomfortable it can feel to begin yet another attempt at weight loss…when those in the past never really worked. Don't worry. We will show you the way.

You may have encountered advice and tips from positive psychology or other forms of self-help. What we've designed here is different: It's a path that is physical, emotional, and mental; one that is backed by the latest neuroscience and research into habit formation, our reward pathways, and getting at the root of addictive behaviors. It's also supported by some of the most advanced research in nutrition and exercise physiology. We take all of the science and bundle it up with some good old-fashioned common sense and real-life experience, and deliver it to you in this guide. Extreme Transformation is real, and it's yours.

THE TRIAXIOM: THREE PRINCIPLES OF EXTREME TRANSFORMATION

While the new Extreme Cycle is a potent combination of high- and low-carb days to give you effective and reliable *weight loss* results, the real secret to lifelong *transformation* is lying underneath the diet. Extreme Transformation is not just about how you eat and how you exercise. It's about changing habits and replacing them with a whole new way of thinking and being. It's rehabilitation.

Over the past few years, we've distilled down our observations of those who have become truly and permanently successful in their weight loss and maintenance, as well as reflections on our own experience, plus a deep dive into the most current research in the areas of integrative nutrition, exercise physiology, and neuroscience. We've simplified everything into three principles that encompass all that we do for people—focusing on their bodies, their hearts, and their minds. For lifelong change and weight loss, no single principle can exist without the others. They all must happen together. You'll feel amazing, and best of all, you'll know how and why you feel amazing.

These three principles consist of 21 lessons, which fall into the three weeks of transformation:

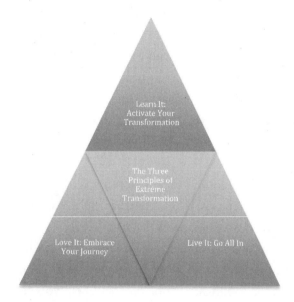

Week One: Learn It

The first seven lessons will teach you what it takes to make the radical shift in thinking that is necessary at the beginning of your journey of transformation. You will dig deep and find two critical components for lifelong change: your *what* and your *why*. You'll identify exactly *what* it is that you want to achieve, and *why*; the motivating factors that will lead you to these goals. Then we will help you discover the true path to transformation that has been there all along. This path is in all of us, but it often lies hidden. Seeing the true path will completely shift our focus off the diet and exercise and place it where it belongs for lifelong change. We then teach you the crucial lessons of setting up your environment and your support system for success, tracking your progress, and best of all—making the journey fun!

The steps in this section will have you rethinking every weight loss program you've ever done. We will show you a path to the lifelong transformation that you have always wanted. It has always been there; you just didn't know how to see it!

Week Two: Love It

In Week Two, you will go from learning the process of Extreme Transformation into mental and emotional action—actually taking the steps toward believing in yourself, your true abilities, and the process that leads directly to success. You will find a place that is honest and vulnerable so that you can peel away all the excuses that you've used in the past. You will learn how to unload the *real* weight—to finally be at peace with any unresolved emotional trauma you have experienced in the past—that is holding you back from living your life to the fullest.

You will take responsibility for your actions, you will learn how to identify and banish the negative self-talk that has held you back, and ultimately embrace a whole new identity—one built on self-love, integrity, and dignity!

Finally, you will address your fears. We know and understand these fears, and we are going to teach you tactics to conquer them once and for all. We'll take you through some tough situations that will help you get inside yourself—maybe to a place that you've never let yourself go before. Don't be afraid.

We have seen it all, and nearly every individual who begins to Love It—embrace their journey with enthusiasm—will tell you that it is one of the greatest accomplishments of their life. In the end, you will feel powerfully free from those chains that have held you back in the past.

Week Three: Live It

The lessons in Week Three prepare you to handle the challenges ahead, and set you up to live a life of transformation. You will learn how to become a priority in your own life, and you will know how to defend your priorities aggressively so that no one will stand in the way of your success. We will lay out inevitable obstacles ahead that will try to derail your progress. When you do fall off track, we will teach you the tried-and-true method to getting right back on. And we will shine a spotlight on your current triggers, so that you can identify them and navigate safely around or through them.

These lessons will help you uproot deeply engrained behaviors that have kept you fixed in patterns of coping with triggers by eating foods that not only add weight, but are most likely making you sick. You will learn how to replace these bad habits, addictions to food, and routines that have been sabotaging you, with a new way of living so that you can continue to lose weight and maintain that weight loss—forever.

Janey's Story

Janey's story has inspired thousands of followers on my blog HeidiPowell.net. Check out how this single mom lost 36 pounds, going from 158 to 122, and got into the best shape of her life!

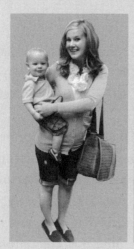 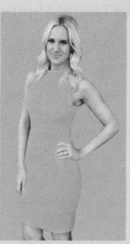

"Health and fitness have not always been my forte. Just a few years ago I couldn't run to the end of my block without feeling winded and the only veggies in my life were the limp celery slices that came with my Buffalo wings. I was over 30 pounds heavier, unhealthy, unhappy, out of shape, *and* freshly divorced. At 21, with a toddler in tow, I was about to start my life over, and just the thought of facing the world after that kind of pain and heartbreak was enough to keep me in bed with only a large cheese pizza to keep me company…seriously, I once ate an entire cheese pizza in an attempt to drown my sorrows! It was time for a change, and the day I signed divorce papers was also the day I committed to leading a healthy lifestyle for the rest of my life. That's when I met Heidi and Chris. I started slow and began to see small changes happening in my body, and I loved it. Just three months after I had made it my goal to change my life, I crossed the finish line of my very first 10K. Best. Feeling. Ever. Ironically, it was on this exact same day that I told my boyfriend (now husband), Kyle, that I loved him for the first time, another huge feat I never imagined possible.

"About a year ago, almost exactly three years after deciding to start my life over, my husband and I crossed off one of the final "to-do's" on my fitness bucket list and completed a half marathon together, crossing the finish line hand in hand. It was so symbolic of all of the changes I had made in my life to get to this point, and was easily one of the most emotionally raw moments of my life. So grateful to have my husband alongside me in this journey!"

IT'S YOUR LIFE. NOW LIVE IT WITH ENTHUSIASM!

Throughout this guide, you will read about and see the amazing transformations we have helped others achieve. The results speak for themselves. We are confident in our methodology because time and time again we have proven firsthand its life-changing power.

The 21 days and their accompanying lessons are crucial to your transformation. They are the stepping-stones to the grander path that you will be achieving and accessing. What you are in for is so much bigger, so much more powerful, so much more fulfilling than anything you've ever imagined. Yes, your weight loss will be amazing and fitness will improve—they are goals that keep on giving and giving. But the empowered heart and clarity of mind that come from understanding and finally appreciating yourself—are priceless.

We're so excited for you.

Now here we go!

Chapter Two

HOW THE EXTREME CYCLE WORKS

During the last three seasons of *Extreme Weight Loss* we used an innovative new approach to carb cycling to see if, as predicted, it would help our people lose their desired weight in a more sustainable way. This cycle, which we call the Extreme Cycle, is made up of five high-carb days, followed by two low-carb days.

This flow worked wonders for all of our participants. They not only lost weight easily and immediately and without feeling rocked by big changes to their eating habits, but also felt strong and stable enough to continue eating this way when they went home after 90 days of boot camp with us and beyond.

As Jeff told us, "Ever since I truly committed to Chris and Heidi's Extreme Cycle, I am finally feeling amazing. I eat something delicious and filling every three hours. I set aside time for myself every day to train—and I want to. I'm seeing results every week. I like who I am and how I feel. I even got a tattoo on my arm that says THIS IS MY LIFE NOW. This experience saved my family and my life."

We are going to share a lot more about Jeff's transformation—his story is an amazing ride of highs and lows and ultimately true transformation (see page 128). But we are sharing his testimonial because we want to give you a sense of just how passionately our participants respond to the Extreme Cycle and how amazing it feels to lose weight with confidence and control.

In a nutshell, we have designed our Extreme Cycle so that it:

- Gives you a way to eat that is convenient, simple, delicious, and satiating.
- Enables you to continuously lose at least one percent of your body weight each week.
- Increases your body awareness (we will explain why this is so important to continued weight loss and commitment to your goals).

So what does this all mean? If you are 5'6" and weigh 275 pounds now, you can lose upwards of seven or more pounds per 21-day cycle; if you weigh 155 pounds at 5'2" you can lose up to five or more pounds per 21-day cycle. Or if you weigh 350 pounds at 6', you can feasibly lose over ten or more pounds per 21-day cycle. And keep in mind, you can accelerate these numbers even more to lose weight as fast as the participants on the show if you choose—we'll show you how. The beauty and brilliance of Extreme Transformation is that once you establish your goals, you can repeat the 21-day cycle for as long as you need to reach them.

The point is that Extreme Transformation is both realistic and successful. It requires changes, but it doesn't wreak havoc on your daily life and make you feel like you have to live in a bubble of deprivation and restriction. You are at home, at work, living your life—*losing weight and getting fit.*

MASTERING YOUR METABOLISM AND CREATING WEIGHT LOSS

The number of calories you burn each day varies according to how active you are. If you follow the same routine every day, eating and moving around (or not) in pretty much the same ways, you'll burn roughly the same number of calories every day. The proportion of calories used by each of your body's three energy consumers—digestion, maintenance, and movement—will also stay pretty constant.

So, how many calories are we talking about? That depends on some factors: your gender, your height, your weight, and your age. Generally, a bigger body needs more calories than a smaller one does, and a younger body needs more calories than an older body does.

All these numbers are swell, but you're reading this book because you want to slim down, not because you want to study science. Let's put the facts and figures together into tools that will help you get the body you want. The arithmetic of weight loss is super-simple:

- Each day that you eat more calories than your metabolism burns, your body stores the extra energy as body fat. You gain weight.
- Eat the same number of calories as your metabolism burns, and your body neither builds nor uses up its stores of fat. You maintain your weight.
- Eat fewer calories than your metabolism burns, and your body makes up the energy shortfall by tapping into your fat. You lose weight. This is what fitness professionals call a *calorie deficit,* and it's the key to weight loss.
- The calorie deficit is what weight loss is all about. If you want to drop the pounds, you have to run your metabolism at a deficit. How big a deficit? Here's the magic number: To lose one pound of fat in a given window of time—say, a week—you've got to burn 3,500 more calories than you take in. That doesn't mean you have to cut out 3,500 calories a day (you probably don't even eat that much!). But to lose weight you do have to eat less. Most carb-cyclers find that they get the best results by creating a 500- to 1,000-calorie deficit through their diet daily—then boost the deficit even more through Accelerators!

Keeping your own metabolism in mind as you work the 21-day cycle is an important tool to keep you focused on your calorie intake. If you begin to plateau, for instance, check in and make sure that your calories didn't spike.

WHAT IS CARB CYCLING?

Carb Cycling is an alternating, patterned way of eating to maximize the ability to manipulate your body for fat loss. High-carb days consist of predominantly high-protein, *high*-carb, low-fat meals. Low-carb days consist of predominantly high-protein, *low*-carb, high-fat meals.

During high-carb days, there is a moderate to high insulin response after the meals, triggering a temporary anabolic state—driving nutrients into the muscles and boosting metabolic rate. During low-carb days, there is a minimal insulin response after the meals, keeping the body in a mostly catabolic state—breaking down and oxidizing fat. Long story short, high-carb days boost your metabolism (while still losing fat), and low-carb days turbocharge your fat loss.

Carb Cycling has actually been used in the fitness industry for decades as a powerful way to positively alter body composition by maximizing fat burn while maintaining muscle mass. With the Extreme Cycle, we just put a real-life twist on it, and the results speak for themselves: Incredible weight loss, eating foods that you enjoy, without crashing your metabolism.☺

WHAT IS THE *EXTREME* CYCLE?

The Extreme Cycle is a continuous pattern of four high-carb days followed by two low-carb days, then a Reset day. Because of the strategic way the high-carb and low-carb days are structured, you lose weight more steadily, and in a way that makes you feel balanced and controlled. You'll learn how to truly manipulate your body to maximize fat loss and turn good numbers on the scale every week. With each passing week, you will feel stronger and more agile. As you integrate the daily Metabolic Missions, you will increase your lean muscle mass and tone your body. When you add the weight loss Accelerators, you'll see the numbers on the scale drop even faster.

Extreme Cycle Weekly Schedule

Here's a broad overview of what a week of the Extreme Cycle looks like:

Day 1: Monday: High-Carb Day

Day 2: Tuesday: High-Carb Day

Day 3: Wednesday: High-Carb Day

Day 4: Thursday: High-Carb Day

Day 5: Friday: Low-Carb Day

Day 6: Saturday: Low-Carb Day

Day 7: Sunday: Weigh-In and Reset Day

How the Extreme Cycle Works on the Inside: The Science

Before we go any further, we feel it's helpful for you to understand how the Extreme Cycle is specifically designed to maximize your weight loss experience—both physically and psychologically.

We're going to drop some science on you here. If you're a physiology and psychology geek like us, then enjoy! ☺ If not, don't worry…we'll break it all down for you in "normal" terms beyond this section. You'll see that there is a specific purpose to every component of the Extreme Cycle design. We developed the cycle this way for a multitude of physiological and psychological reasons:

1. The calorie ranges are designed so that for six days of the week you will be in an overall calorie deficit—which means that the body will spend more time breaking down fat stores (mobilizing) and using them for energy (oxidizing). As long as the calorie deficit is maintained, the laws of physics remain on your side—and always work. When you consume less energy than your body burns, you lose weight. That's the beauty of physics. Even on high-carb days, the total of your meals is designed to result in a calorie deficit, so you will consistently lose weight. On low-carb days, the weight loss process is turbocharged even more.

2. Starting with four high-carb days in a row gives a type of "normalcy" to a structured way of eating every day. It creates mental comfort and allows you to get into

a groove with meals and preferences that work for you. Alternating between high- and low-carb days is effective, but switching between days can be confusing and disruptive to our habitual patterns. The beauty and ease of this Extreme Carb Cycle pattern allows for the powerful nature of carb cycling, without the discomfort of significantly uprooting your eating patterns.

3. Carbs are *necessary* for weight loss! Carbohydrates are the "92-octane fuel" that powers our brain, our muscles, and the rest of the organs of our body. Fueling the body with carbs puts more fuel into the muscles, yielding greater intensity and effort during workouts—which then results in a greater metabolic afterburn (more calories burned at rest) and stronger stimulus for muscle development and growth.

4. Carbs in the diet are directly linked to more effective thyroid conversion in the liver—therefore keeping metabolic rate up. Low-carb diets blunt thyroid conversion and ultimately result in metabolic slowdown. Four high-carb days in a row get the metabolic furnace burning red-hot, priming the body for maximum fat loss when switching over to the low-carb days.

5. Breakfast always includes a carbohydrate and a fat—in addition to a protein—for a couple of reasons. The carbohydrates are designed to replace liver glycogen lost during the overnight fast (glycogen was used to fuel the heartbeat and diaphragm during sleep). Since the liver is one of the main controlling organs of the body, filling up its store of glycogen puts the body into a "fed" state—which essentially signals the body to "wake up" and increase metabolic processes. The fats are designed to slow digestion, keeping you fuller well into the morning and just in time for your midmorning snack (meal 2).

6. Starchy carbohydrates are a no-no at dinner. While there are still carbs included in the form of fibrous vegetables (leafy greens or cruciferous veggies), all sugars and starches are out. This is to prevent a rise in blood sugar in the evening. Instead, by pulling starchy and sugary carbs, the body is more likely to have a minor insulin response, remaining in a catabolic state into the overnight fast, which keeps your body mobilizing (breaking down) and oxidizing (burning) fat well into the night...when the body experiences a metabolic slowdown. Basically, when done right, you don't store fat at night this way—you actually burn it while you are sleeping!

7. After four high-carb days, we drop into two low-carb days. This is where the *real* control over your weight loss starts to take place. Pulling carbs from your meals and snacks flips the switch to turbocharge

the rate at which your body burns fat. However, because you don't have starchy carbs in your system, your body does not release as much insulin, triggering your body to burn fat instead—you go into maximized fat mobilization and oxidation.

8. The two low-carb days are also designed to help remove any excess water retention and bloating in the body. Starchy carbs are like magnets for water. Therefore, removing sugary and starchy carbs from the diet for two days results in a natural release of water—revealing a more true weight on the scale.

Imagine being a sculptor in this process. You put a light blanket of water over your body during the four high-carb days. During this time you chisel away under the blanket with good nutrition, Metabolic Missions, and Accelerators—carving the body you want. After four days, you drop into two low-carb days, pulling the blanket off and revealing the progress so far. The next week you do it again...and again...each week putting the blanket over the sculpture and working away, revealing the latest results every weigh-in...until you are finally finished with your masterpiece.

This is the beauty of the Extreme Cycle and makes you the true artist here. You're in total control the whole way!

9. Every seventh day, you will weigh yourself in the morning, then reset your metabolism, rest your body, and give yourself a reward. Physiologically, the increase in calories boosts metabolism significantly. Psychologically, the Reset day gives us something to look forward to, so we don't feel deprived on this journey. This is your chance to satisfy any cravings you may have, relieving any feelings of restriction. On Reset days, you eat high-carb meals and snacks, but you can also reward yourself with a Clean Cheat snack or meal (see page 86 for a complete list of Clean Cheats). Rest and reward are a huge part of avoiding feelings of deprivation and preventing overwhelming cravings.

So there you have it: a broad overview of *how* the Extreme Cycle works to help you reach your weight loss goals quickly and comfortably.

As you will soon see, we have designed the 21-day cycle so that your meal planning is fast and enjoyable. We've laid it all out for you with quick-and-easy recipes. In fact, several of these recipes were inspired by gourmet chef David Rushing, who lost over 200 pounds during Season 4 of *Extreme Weight Loss*. Through his journey of transformation, he took his extensive knowledge of the culinary arts and weight loss experience, and helped us to create many of the delectable meals you will enjoy in this book!

We've also provided simple, go-to meal suggestions, and a three-step plan to creating your own meals if you don't want to bother with the recipes. Those are all listed on page 72.

WHAT DO I EAT?

Contrary to popular belief that we need to restrict certain nutrients to lose weight and to nourish our bodies for optimum weight loss, we need *all* of the main macronutrients—proteins, carbohydrates, *and* fats. The secret is in how we combine them in our meals to manipulate our bodies to do what we want them to do—lose fat!

In order to create the powerful meal combinations in the Extreme Cycle, we must categorize foods into different macronutrients based upon their predominant nutrient content. For example, lean ground turkey is predominantly made of protein; however, it may have 2 or 3 grams of fat. Therefore, lean ground turkey falls into the protein category. Most foods are not exclusively *one* macronutrient, but have trace amounts of other macros in them. We have done all of the footwork for you, and have categorized them for the most effective meal combinations!

Protein

Protein is vital to the proper functioning of our muscles, brain, organs, and other tissues, and is the foundation macronutrient used in the Extreme Cycle. We eat it with every meal. Protein is the building block for the most active metabolic tissues of our body—our muscles—and we need to make sure they are nourished with every meal. In addition, protein is a quickly satiating nutrient, meaning that it makes us full when we eat it. Because of this, we prefer to eat protein first at every meal to make us immediately full. It's a quick and easy rule that we have used for years, and it works like a charm to curb cravings and prevent overeating carbs or fats later!

Some of the proteins you will enjoy include:

- Protein shakes and smoothies
- Lean beef
- Fat-free and low-fat dairy such as cottage cheese, Greek yogurt, and egg whites
- Chicken, turkey, and pork tenderloin
- Fish and shellfish
- Soy protein sources such as tofu and tempeh
- Other vegetarian protein options such as hemp, bean, and pea protein
- And many more…check out Appendix D for the full list!

Carbohydrates

Carbohydrates have been demonized over the past couple decades as a main cause of the obesity epidemic, but when you eat the right carbs at the right times, they can actually be one of your greatest allies in the weight loss battle. All carbs are broken down into the sugar called glucose—which is the high-octane fuel our cells are designed to function on. In short, carbs nourish our body! When we get the right amount of glucose in our system, it nourishes our liver, our muscles, our brain, and all of our other organs. It naturally boosts our metabolism and primes our body for maximum weight loss. In fact, there's a saying in the physiology world that "fat burns in a carbohydrate fire."

However, too much glucose in our system is not a good thing. That's why when losing weight we want to avoid carbohydrates that are broken down quickly in our system. These carbs are the highly processed, starchy, or sugary carbs found in snacks, junk foods, or baked goods. Instead, when following the Extreme Cycle, we nourish our body regularly with quality carbs that are broken down slowly, to trickle the glucose into our bloodstream. These are the real, clean, natural carbohydrates found in foods like:

- Whole grains (rice, breads, pastas, cereals, popcorn)
- Beans and legumes

- Root vegetables (potatoes, yams, squash, et cetera)
- Fruit

(A full list of all the healthy foods is in Appendix D.)

These carbs are packed with vitamins and minerals, high in fiber, and digested easily by your body so that it feels satisfied, and you feel energetic.

While protein is mandatory at each meal, there is an optional food on the Extreme Cycle that you can add to, or remove from your meals, based upon your customized needs—vegetables! Whereas vegetables are technically a carbohydrate, most are rich in fiber and extremely low in any calorie impact. Because of this, we classify these in their own special category and consider them a so-called "free food": They can be enjoyed in limitless portions, and are one of the most powerful tools for feeling full and satiated.

Veggies are high in fiber, water, and valuable antioxidants, and we highly advise you to eat as many as possible in your meals—although it is not mandatory. We make veggies an optional food because oftentimes the amount of mandatory food you are already eating in your meals can have such volume, it can be difficult to consume so much food. However, if you struggle with cravings, adding veggies to your meals will be an incredibly powerful tactic to curb any cravings and keep you feeling full and satisfied throughout the day.

We're going to show you some amazing ways to volumize your meals to gigantic proportions using delicious vegetables. Follow our list of veggies, and they're yours to enjoy in limitless amounts. You are approved to eat all the veggies you want—anytime!

- Broccoli
- Cauliflower
- Green beans
- Carrots
- Onions
- Spinach
- And many more…

Fats

Fats are the third main macronutrient—and a powerful one at that! Our brains rely on fats—especially the essential fatty acids such as omega-3s and omega-6s—to maintain proper cellular function and hormonal balance. These fats are enormously important to how our brain and bodies manage the hormones that regulate our body temperature, our moods, and our digestion.

However, following the Extreme Cycle, we use fats to trick your body and your mind to make weight loss SO much easier. Fats have a powerful effect on slowing digestion and keeping our stomachs full. When we use the right fats at the right time, we can curb cravings and maximize fat loss at the same time. Keep reading and we'll show you how!

Often people worry when they think about cutting out carbs for two days, but adding in some tasty fats *really* opens up the food options for delicious meals! Check out the kinds of dietary fats you can have on these low-carb days. You're going to start looking forward to these days!

- Egg yolk
- Butter
- Heavy Cream
- Cheese
- Bacon
- Olives
- Avocado
- Nuts and seeds
- Olive and flaxseed oil
- Nut butters such as peanut butter and almond butter
- And many more...

As you can see, you will be eating an array of delicious, enjoyable foods. Just wait until you see the meals and recipes we lay out for you—it only gets better! Now, let's take a look at the different meal combinations we use following the Extreme Cycle, to maximize your fat loss results:

BREAKFAST:
IGNITE YOUR DAY

Our parents were right. Breakfast really *is* the most important meal of the day. It helps "*break* the *fast*" from not eating for many hours, and helps jump-start your metabolism from its overnight slumber (slowdown). No matter whether it is a high- or a low-carb day, your breakfast breakdown is always the same: Protein + Carbohydrate + Fats.

High-Carb Days

After breakfast things change a little bit:

For Meals 2, 3, and 4 on high-carb days, you will be eating carbohydrates with each meal and cutting out the dietary fats, so it looks like this:

For Meal 5 on a high-carb day, we will remove the carbohydrate and replace it with a healthy fat to flip the fat-burning switch. It will look like this:

Low-Carb Days

After breakfast on the low-carb days, we cut carbs and instead eat fats with each of the last 4 meals, so it looks like this:

Reset Days

Once a week on your weigh-in day, you get to reset your metabolism and reward yourself for a job well done! Your Reset day is neither a high-carb nor a high-fat day…it's more of a high-*calorie* day. Reset day is incredibly important for a few reasons: Physiologically, the increase in calories boosts your metabolic rate for more effective fat loss the following days. Mentally, it satisfies any psychological or emotional cravings that you may be experiencing, so that you will never feel deprived and risk straying from your weight loss journey. We have even designed some incredible Clean Cheat recipes (see page 269) to help you bump up your calories for your Reset day, while indulging in some of your favorite delicacies. However, instead of cheap junk food, you'll be eating high-quality foods that will nourish your body and prepare you for the best weight loss results. Some of these recipes include:

- Hootenanny Pancakes
- BLT Burger and Sweet Potato Fries
- Barbecue Chicken Pita Pizza
- Spinach Artichoke Dip
- Peanut Butter Chocolate Chip Cookie Dough
- Mac and Cheese with Bacon
- And *many* more...

As you can see, there is a *lot* to look forward to with this program. You are in for some delicious new dishes. Who said dieting had to be bland?!

WHEN DO I EAT?

With the Extreme Carb Cycle, you will be eating every three hours. Think of your metabolism as a furnace for your body. Eat less often and your metabolism cools down; eat more often and it heats up. The hotter your furnace gets, the more fuel it burns, including the stored fat that hasn't been doing anything but weighing you down!

Following the Extreme Cycle, we always eat breakfast within 30 minutes of waking, then eat a meal every three hours after. A typical Extreme Cycle meal schedule (whether high-carb or low-carb) looks like this:

Wake up at 6:30 a.m.
Meal 1: Breakfast at 7:00 a.m.

Meal 2: Morning snack at 10:00 a.m.
Meal 3: Lunch at 1:00 p.m.
Meal 4: Afternoon snack at 4:00 p.m.
Meal 5: Dinner at 7:00 p.m.

Of course, you would adjust this schedule depending on when you wake up. If you are a very early riser, you might be starting your breakfast at 6:00 a.m. and finishing your dinner around 6:00 p.m. Even if you work the midnight shift and wake up at 7:00 p.m. every day, the rules still apply: Eat within 30 minutes of waking and approximately every three hours thereafter!

Reality Check

Look, we know that life has all kinds of unexpected twists and turns, especially when it comes to the daily grind. The timing of your meals does not have to be *exactly* every three hours; just try to get it as close as possible. Sometimes you may eat every two and a half hours, sometimes every four hours. If your days run long and you find yourself hungry after your final meal, try spacing out your meals to every three and a half hours, so you eat closer to the time you go to bed. With the Extreme Cycle, *you* create the meal timing that works best in your life!

WATER, WATER, WATER

We cannot stress enough the importance of drinking a *lot* of water when on the weight loss journey. Fact of the matter is that if you don't drink enough water, you will not lose the weight at your fastest potential. Why? Water is the main ingredient in the majority of the metabolic processes of the body—which is the driving force behind weight loss! Proper hydration keeps metabolism high, increases mental clarity and energy, and is a powerful influencer for curbing cravings. In addition, living the Extreme Transformation lifestyle, you will be exercising more, so you will lose fluids faster through perspiration and breathing, making hydration even more important.

Did you know that nearly 90 percent of Americans are chronically dehydrated? And unfortunately, most of us go through our days without realizing it, causing us to suffer from unnecessary fatigue and increased cravings. Early on your journey, we are going to ask you to drink an extra quart of water every day. However, ultimately we would like you to work up to drinking at least a gallon of water every day. This will be critical in maximizing your results!

Take the Hydration Test

Pinch the skin on the back of your hand and let go. If your skin stays puckered for any length of time then you are more than likely dehydrated. Also, keep an eye on your urine. If the color is slightly yellow or darker, your body is telling you that it needs fluid. And since water is the safest fluid, we suggest sticking to drinking water. Drink until your urine is consistently clear or just slightly yellow. Then you'll know your body's hydration is primed for fat loss!

Reality Check

Let's get real. Like many of you, we don't like to drink regular water. It is bland, especially when trying to push a gallon or more every day! If we're going to get that much water in, we need to *want* to drink it. We need flavor! There are some *amazing* low- and no-calorie sweeteners out there for water these days. Feel free to grab some (or a lot) at the supermarket, and flavor away to stay well hydrated during your transformation journey. Carry a huge water bottle around with you every day (from 1 liter to 1 gallon), flavored however you choose!

Chris Tip

To make sure you get all the water you need, follow our 10-gulp rule:

Every time the water bottle touches your lips, take 10 gulps before putting it down... and you will stay well hydrated all day long!

Heidi Tip
Vitamins, Minerals, and Fiber

Even though following the Extreme Cycle will have you eating highly nutritious foods, anytime you are eating fewer calories than you are burning, your body is most likely at a slight deficit in its necessary vitamins, minerals, and fiber as well. You may want to supplement the Extreme Cycle with a good multivitamin to make sure your body is getting the vitamins and minerals it needs to perform at its best. In addition, we recommend adding at least 1 tablespoon of psyllium fiber to your daily meals (it's usually added to a protein shake or some other liquid) to ensure proper fiber intake. A healthy body begins with a healthy gut—which is where all of our nutrients are absorbed! Fiber is nature's "scrub brush" for the intestines; if you add at least an extra tablespoon of fiber daily, your body and bowels will thank you for it!

HOW MUCH DO I EAT?

Any weight loss plan inevitably begs the question: How much do I eat if I want to lose weight? Science dictates that fat is lost only when we take in fewer calories than our body burns. A lot of different plans use different methods to accomplish this goal: points, portion plates, hand portions, pre-planned recipes, and so on. In previous books, we taught quick-and-easy portion sizing using your hand as a measure. While this works for most people in reducing their calorie intake and teaches appropriate portions, Extreme Cycling is a precision program. Yes, all of the recipes are dialed in to maximize your weight loss, but we are going to show you what's happening behind the curtain—so that you have the power to create your own meal combinations, and customize your own menu if you choose!

We have designed our calorie guidelines and portion sizes to work for most people who are seeking to optimize the way they feel during the days, and optimize the weight they see on the scale every week. In most cases, the recipes are tailored for women at 1,500 calories, and 2,000 calories for men—in our experience, these are typical calorie allotments that enable weight loss and quick-and-easy troubleshooting when combined with an exercise plan. In general, men tend to have more muscle mass, so they are allotted more calories than women. You will want to pay attention to these calorie differences when you prepare your meals and follow the recipes. All the recipes contain adjustments for men and women.

Chris Tip

You will find that even though we talk about eating low dietary fat on high-carb days, it is impossible to go a full day without eating at least *some* dietary fats. You actually need some fat every day for proper metabolic function, and fats are bound to be present, even in low-fat, high-carbohydrate foods. That's why typically on a high-carb day, around 20 percent of your calories consumed will come incidentally from dietary fat.

Same goes for low-carb days. Carbohydrates are going to occur naturally in some of your foods—much of them as fiber on these days—but still there will be some light starches that may find their way into your meals to the tune of about 20 or so percent. Not to worry. The structure is designed for this.

Just as with everything in life—*nothing* is perfect. You are not expected to hit these exact numbers for every meal. You'll even see that the recipes we have designed for you don't hit the numbers perfectly—but overall they come darn close. With most things in life, "close enough" doesn't cut it. So be grateful that this diet is so beautifully structured that as long as you come close on your portions, you win.

Quick Meals on the Go

Realistically speaking, we know that you will not always have a chance to prepare your own meals. When you find yourself eating elsewhere, a quick-and-easy rule of thumb to get close to appropriate portions for you would be to follow the hand-portion guide:

Proteins: Palm-size portion
Grainy, starchy carbs & fruit: 1 clenched fist
Veggie carbs: 2 clenched fists
Fats: 1 thumb
Sauces: 1 thumb

Josh's Story

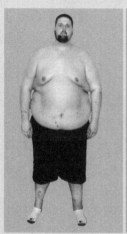 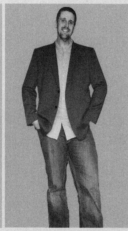

Josh tried out for *Extreme Weight Loss* but did not make the cut. At 6'9" he had gained 300 pounds, tipping the scales at 585 pounds at only 25 years old. Not being selected for the show, however, was just the beginning of Josh's transformation story. He was so committed to his own process that he buckled down and did the Extreme Cycle on his own. Within a year, he had lost 233 pounds. As he described, "I was so unhappy. I knew that this life wasn't the one I imagined. I stopped talking to girls. I stopped going out with my friends. I was a shut-in—always so sick and tired. I realized that I didn't need the TV show to make the change. And in the very first week, I lost 26 pounds. I never looked back."

Josh said that learning the Extreme Cycle and eating every three hours "just worked. I never ever felt hungry. I didn't have to ever feel deprived. Eating like this is now just second nature." Josh has now lost over 300 pounds and is currently a personal trainer, helping others achieve their dreams of living happy and healthy lives.

Know this: As soon as you switch to the Extreme Cycle, your brain and body awareness will reconnect, and your hormonal signals will right themselves. Extreme Cycling is a livable, convenient, satisfying way to eat. You won't feel like you're dieting or depriving yourself, but instead you'll feel like an artist, sculpting your new body each week under total control. Designing your meals for weight loss, eating every three hours, and drinking adequate amounts of water will open your eyes to a whole new quality of life.

Onward and upward!

Chapter Three

METABOLIC MISSIONS AND ACCELERATORS

The Extreme Cycle nutrition lays down the foundation for your weight loss, but it's exercise that accelerates the results: Exercise is how you control the throttle of your weight loss journey. If you choose, you can lose weight slowly over time with just the Extreme Cycle alone. However, if you want to speed up your weight loss and nearly double your results, then you'll want to add in daily movement to see your body change faster than ever. When you exercise regularly—even if it's only 5 or 15 minutes a day—you stimulate your body's muscles, hormones, and other systems to incinerate more calories. That's why nutrition controls the fat-burning switch—and exercise turbocharges it! And with our Metabolic Missions and Accelerators, we are going to show you how we get our participants to drop extraordinary amounts of weight in record time. Now it's your turn!

WHAT METABOLIC MISSIONS DO FOR YOU

We have designed 15 different Metabolic Missions to be completed during your 21 days of Extreme Transformation. Each Metabolic Mission is a short-duration, high-intensity circuit, designed for maximum metabolic afterburn, as well as to stimulate the muscles for shape and development. As you know, your body is made to move—to push, pull, squat, crunch, run, and jump! So all of the exercises in the missions reflect those basic, natural movements your body is meant to do.

The high-intensity nature of each Metabolic Mission elicits a strong neuro-endocrine response—to release catecholamines, increase oxygen uptake, increase lactic acid in the body, and raise body temperature. Sounds like a lot of blah, blah, science stuff…but this is why it's so awesome: When you train hard and fast, your brain is stimulated to increase the release of growth hormone—this stuff is like liquid gold. Growth hormone is one of the most lipolytic (fat-burning) hormones in the human body, and increases the rate at which the cells replenish themselves. So basically, high-intensity exercise increases fat loss and makes you look and feel younger. Doing the Metabolic Missions is the true path to the fountain of youth!

The Metabolic Missions don't require any equipment and can be done anywhere—at home, in a gym, and outside—whatever works in *your* life and is enjoyable for you! Now, these Metabolic Missions might seem simple, but that doesn't mean they aren't going to test your mettle. These rapid challenges will raise your heart rate, make your muscles burn, and get you the results you want—a slender, more toned body. An added benefit? Once you do them, you help your body burn even *more* calories throughout the day!

The Metabolic Missions are totally scalable by ability and can be done by anyone—whether you haven't worked out in 10 years, or you're already a gym rat. As long as you push yourself, you will take your fitness to new levels.

And to make this process even more forgiving, if you are just starting, you can cut the Metabolic Missions in half until you feel ready to take on a full mission.

Metabolic Mission Code

For our Metabolic Missions, we use five different types of challenges. Each day of the work week (Monday through Friday, or whatever five days work in your schedule), you will embark upon one of these missions…and will not stop until the mission is accomplished!

1. **Stepladders**—These are circuits that either ascend or descend in repetitions. With the ascending stepladders, it's fun to see how far you can get in an allotted amount of time. The descending ladders are awesome because as you progress, the rep counts get smaller and you see an end in sight!

2. **RFT**—This acronym stands for "rounds for time." See how long it takes you to do a set number of rounds of the prescribed circuit!

3. **Chipper**—These circuits have a *lot* of reps of each exercise. It can seem daunting at first, but rep after rep you will "chip away" at the total circuit. See how long it takes to complete one round of the entire circuit!

4. **AMRAP**—This acronym stands for "as many rounds as possible." Whenever you see AMRAP next to a Metabolic Mission, do as many rounds of the circuit in the allotted time as you can!

5. **Tabata**—Tabata was developed by a brilliant physiologist from Japan. It indicates a four-minute exercise routine in which you perform as many repetitions of an exercise as possible for 20 seconds, then take a 10-second rest, then begin again with another 20-second round, followed by a 10-second rest, until you reach four minutes (8 rounds total). When you see Tabata next to one or more exercises, you know what to do: Just Tabata each of the exercises in the list for an amazing workout!

NOTE: Each Mission is a competition, either with yourself or with others. As with any game, it is important to have movement standards—ways to measure if the rep counts! For all of the Metabolic Mission Movements and their competition standards, refer to the detailed instructions in Part Four.

ACCELERATORS

Following the Extreme Cycle and doing Metabolic Missions alone will put you on the path to steady, sustainable weight loss and greater fitness. However, many folks want faster results. We understand. When working with our participants during a one-year transformation, we have 365 days to get these individuals to lose between 100 and 300 pounds. So to accelerate the process and give them the results we all want, we add an Accelerator to their daily program. An Accelerator is a cardio-based exercise or activity that, when added to your normal routine, will aggressively burn body fat and accelerate weight loss. Accelerators are not super-quick high-intensity circuits like the Metabolic Missions. They are activities that raise and maintain an elevated heart rate, that last longer than the missions, and are much less intense. So if you want to accelerate your weight loss, add an Accelerator such as walking, running, soccer, racquetball, biking, or swimming into your routine six days of the week.

An Accelerator keeps your muscles moving and raises your heart rate for a prolonged period of time. The concept is pretty simple: The longer you move, the more calories you burn. Here's the best part about Accelerators: You get to choose the one that works best for you. It can be anything from basketball to rowing, hiking to mixed martial arts. The only major rule is that it has to be fun! If a fun exercise seems far-fetched right now, then for the time being, choose the *most* fun way you can think of to move your body…or maybe something you've always wanted to do. We have no doubt that over time as you begin to explore the capabilities of your body, you really will find *fun* in these activities! We've created a go-to guide to help you find the best Accelerator for you in Lesson 6—Make It Your Own!

What's the most effective Accelerator for fat loss? The quick-and-easy answer is running. You don't have to run *fast*…just run. If you can't run, then jog. If you can't jog, then walk. In our history of extreme transformations, those who began running, jogging, or walking (or any combo of the three), dropped the most weight, the fastest.

However, when it comes to the *best* Accelerator for you, the correct answer is: the one you love to do the most! You have freedom to choose in this journey. If you don't love running, jogging, or walking, then select a fun Accelerator that you love to do!

For those starting out, you will want to ease into your Accelerators. This slow start is done for a multitude of reasons. In the beginning, less is more. If your body has not been exposed to exercise for a long period of time, simply doing a Metabolic Mission and five minutes of Accelerating is more than enough to get some stellar results! But even more important, it's about learning to carve out that time for *you* during the day. Make sure that you can set that daily appointment and keep that promise to yourself every day. (You will read more about putting yourself first in Lesson 17—Be Beneficially Selfish.)

If you want to jump right into an hour-long class or a competitive sports league, then go for it. However, if you are starting out with an individual exercise like walking, jogging, running, rowing, cycling, and so on, you will begin your Accelerator with just 5 minutes. You'll do 5 minutes the first week, then add 5 more minutes for the second week. Then add 5 more minutes for the third. If at *any* time you feel you are unable to increase the duration of your Accelerators, stick with the current duration until you are ready to add the next 5 minutes. It is more important that you keep your commitment to completing a *shorter* period of time rather than commit to accelerating for longer and not do it! Again, we'll go into those very important commitments soon. ☺ In the meantime, here's an idea for how we structure Accelerators for Extreme Transformation:

Intensity	Time spent breaking a sweat (120 bpm minimum)*		
Cycle 1	Week 1: 5 minutes	Week 2: 10 minutes	Week 3: 15 minutes
Cycle 2	Week 4: 20 minutes	Week 5: 25 minutes	Week 6: 30 minutes
Cycle 3	Week 7: 35 minutes	Week 8: 40 minutes	Week 9: 45 minutes
Cycle 4	Week 10: 50 minutes	Week 11: 55 minutes	Week 12: 60 minutes
*To take HR, take pulse (on neck or wrist) for 6 seconds and multiply by 10.			

Please know that this schedule is what it would look like in a perfect world. In reality, an individual may start off doing 5 minutes and remain at 5 minutes for several weeks until he or she is *ready* to move up to 10 minutes. And again, be realistic—this increase in duration may not happen for a while. It may take several 21-day Extreme Transformation cycles to hit 25 or 30 minutes daily—it is all about how much time you are willing to commit to yourself and your health. As your Accelerators get longer, feel free to split them into two or even three different bouts of exercise, if it is more convenient for you.

For our one-year transformations, we encourage our peeps to aim for at least 60 minutes of daily Accelerators starting off, and ultimately they increase to 90 to 120 minutes every day (split into 45- to 60-minute bouts each)! How much weight you want to lose, and how fast you want to lose it…are up to you!!

Make Accelerators Fun with Intervals!

"Cardio sucks." "I hate running." "It's so boring." We've heard it all, and we understand. Heck, we sometimes feel the same way. But what if cardio was actually fun and entertaining, and the time flew by? When sports are your Accelerators, it's pretty easy to get wrapped up in the game…but how can we make those individual sports like jogging, running, rowing, and cycling more entertaining? Intervals! Not only do they break up the monotony of steady-state cardio, they actually burn fat at an even faster rate—both during and after the bout of exercise! Any Accelerator can quickly pass when you're chipping away with these high- and low-intensity challenges! We use five different intervals for our peeps:

Thrilling Thirties: :30 low intensity / :30 high-intensity

Mighty Minutes: 1:00 low intensity / 1:00 high-intensity

Nasty Nineties: 1:30 low intensity / 1:30 high-intensity

Tenacious Twos: 2:00 low intensity / 2:00 high-intensity

Dirty Two-Thirties: 2:30 low intensity / 2:30 high-intensity

For example, if you're jogging and doing "Mighty Minutes," you will slow to a walk/jog for 60 seconds, then speed up to fast jogging/running for 60 seconds, then slow back down to the walk/jog for 60 seconds, then speed back up for 60 seconds. Repeat until your Accelerator duration is completed! The high and low intensity is completely up to you, but be sure to challenge yourself and don't let your heart rate drop below 120 beats per minute (bpm) during the low-intensity intervals!

Most of our peeps love these intervals that we do; however, some prefer to play with other interval types, like:

- Playlist intervals: One song high-intensity, one song low intensity
- Distance intervals: One lap around the block fast, one lap slow—or walk to one light post, run to the next, etc.

No matter how you interval, you win!

During the 21 days, we will prescribe different intervals each day for you to play with.

Check out Step 6: Make It Your Own! for other fun ways to accelerate your weight loss and get phenomenal results!

HOW AND WHEN TO DO YOUR METABOLIC MISSIONS AND ACCELERATORS

When to Exercise

We both prefer to wake up in the morning and do our workout right away. It's a great way to start the day, plus the majority of the calories you eat after exercise will be partitioned into repairing and building muscle. In addition, the high-intensity Metabolic Mission spikes metabolism for hours afterward, so your body will continue to burn calories at a faster rate than it would without exercise. Most important, and we're sure this will resonate with many of you, we have four kids. Life gets busy really quickly around our home. Most days, if it doesn't happen first thing in the morning, it doesn't happen at all!

But here's the deal. *Any* time you can find to exercise is a "win" in our book. If you can't exercise first thing in the morning, find a time that you trust in your schedule and stick to it. That's the main point: Carve out that time for you every day—and do it. Regardless of whether you train in the morning or at night, as long as you *train*, you are going to get phenomenal results!

Heidi Tip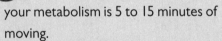

We are all too busy to work out, but part of your new transformation lifestyle is finding time every day to move your body. Here are two of my favorite—and most popular—tips for carving out time to work out:

1. Wake up 15 minutes earlier than you normally do. Not an hour, not even 30 minutes. All it takes to jump-start your metabolism is 5 to 15 minutes of moving.

2. Take advantage of nap time! For those of you who are moms with little kids, when it's time for the little people to sleep, it's time for you to move! And if the kids don't nap, let them join in. My two youngest love nothing more than to follow me around, imitating my workout!

Days to Exercise

We've designed a full schedule of Metabolic Missions and Accelerators into your 21-day sequence of Extreme Transformation. We do Metabolic Missions and Accelerators on Days 1 through 5 of each week, and do an extra Accelerator on Day 6—to maximize your weigh-in on Day 7. It is critically important that you do not work out every day of the week. You *must* have a rest day. Five days of Metabolic Missions and six days of Accelerators will put some physical stress on the body—and it needs at least one day to rest, recover, and reset itself for the week ahead!

When to Eat

If you train in the morning, there are several ways to eat around your Metabolic Mission. If you have an iron stomach, feel free to eat beforehand. However, if you find yourself a bit queasy working out on a full stomach, either eat half your breakfast before and half after, or simply eat breakfast when the mission is complete.

As you will soon see, the 21-day plan in the pages ahead is set up so you can simply follow the Extreme Cycle nutrition, Metabolic Mission, and Accelerator described for each day.

Summary: The Five Rules of Extreme Transformation

To sum it all up, here are the Extreme Transformation five rules of weight loss—the key to taking control of your metabolism so that you can lose the weight you want and keep it off forever:

1. Eat within 30 minutes of waking and every 3 hours after.

2. Follow the Extreme Cycle daily meal combinations.

3. Drink lots of water all day long.

4. Build muscle and spike your metabolism through Metabolic Missions 5 days a week.

5. Accelerate your weight loss daily through fun cardio options 6 days a week.

PART 2

21 Days
to Extreme
Transformation

WARNING: Transformation is an active physical, mental, and emotional process.

Each of the 21 days has an adjoining lesson with psychological and emotional activities that will help you lay down daily habits and create the mental awareness to keep the weight off forever. From learning the shortcuts of effective meal prep to identifying what your motivating force is, your level of involvement with these lessons will absolutely reflect your potential for long-term success. We highly advise you to focus on these lessons and follow through with the mental activities. They are simple and take very little time, but they provide you with the tools to make a radical shift in your life.

Knowing the path of transformation and having realistic expectations for the journey ahead is critical to your success. Before beginning the journey, we advise you to read, or at least skim, through the following 21 days so that you can see what lies ahead for you. You will find that many of the steps are intertwined and work off each other. Many of the lessons in the later days may be helpful to your journey *now*, so don't feel like you must wait until later in the process to complete the lessons. Read ahead. You can do one a day, or do them all today. There may be information in Day 4 that is pertinent to the beginning of your journey now. Or perhaps Day 17 is a chapter that you need to review on a regular basis to help you move forward with your life. Whatever works for you. This is your journey.

This book is written to be your guide. Don't just go over the lessons and be done with them. They are here to read and re-read…to practice for the rest of your life.

As you embark upon the day-to-day nutrition and exercise components of the next 21 days, review the lesson for that day, revisit it, and re-explore that area of your life and mind further. It will anchor you in your transformation—forever.

POWELL

LEARN IT!

You are here: at a momentous time and place in your life. You are at the beginning of a journey that will change your life forever.

The first seven days of Extreme Transformation are all about learning how to embrace the process and make it yours. You get to be the artist here. Over the next seven days you will identify what *you* want, discover *your* real why, learn how to set *your* goals, and discover a path within *yourself* that you never knew existed. You will learn the importance of keeping commitments to yourself—one promise at a time. You will learn how to customize your nutrition and exercise—so that they work for you—and you will put together your Transformation Team to rally you along the way. These early lessons are critical to getting a feel for how this process truly works. Before beginning this first week, we highly encourage you to read these first seven lessons ahead of time so you are well prepared starting out.

Oh, and last but not least, have fun. ☺

This is going to be awesome!

DAY 1

Before You Begin

Before Day 1 (or the morning of), do your first weigh-in. Record your weight in a daily tracker, in your journal, or on your smartphone. (You will also find a 21-Day Daily Tracker in Appendix A, which you can use as well.)

Chris Tip
Take Your Before Pictures
and Memorialize This Moment

One of the most wonderful gifts you can give yourself during this transformation is *proof of progression*. Not only will this memorialize where exactly you came from (serving as a constant reminder never to go back), but it also will give you a more objective perspective of your own body—so you can see the true results. Naturally, our eyes play tricks on us—*what we see in the mirror is not reality. What we see in pictures is much more objective!* Remember that these pics are just for *you*—unless, of course, you want to share them. And trust us, when this journey is over, these pics will give you some major bragging rights!

Here are a few photo pointers to help you out:

Tip 1—Wear clothing that will give you a *full* view of your body so you can see where the transformation is happening! Since you will be the only one seeing these, *shorts* and a *sports bra* may do the trick for you. You'll want to see your shoulders, arms, abdomen, thighs, and calves.

Tip 2—Snap shots from a few different angles—we personally prefer a front shot and a side/profile shot.

Tip 3—Take a beginning picture and *weekly front and side* pictures after that. You won't be able to see the changes on a day-to-day basis, but when the weekly pictures are lined up, you will be *amazed* at the transformation you are achieving. Use these pictures as *daily reminders* by placing printed copies of the pictures in a visible spot. Try inside your fridge, on your bathroom mirror, in your room, or in the bottom of a drawer that you use often. And if you're *really* proud to show them off, use one as your screensaver!

For your convenience, we have included weekly shopping lists for the delicious recipes in this book (see Appendix B). You'll notice there are separate lists for men and women to help you determine the amount of food *you* will need. Clean Cheat shopping lists are also included there, but we recommend NOT purchasing these foods until the day before Reset day to help keep temptation out of the house throughout the week.

Day 1: High-Carb Day

Meal 1: Breakfast
>   Recipe: Cinnamon French Toast

Meal 2: High-Carb Meal
>   Recipe: Chocolate Peanut Butter and
Banana Smoothie

Meal 3: High-Carb Meal
>   Recipe: Three-Bean Salad with Chicken and Kale

Meal 4: High-Carb Meal
>   Recipe: Sweet Potato Chips, Celery Sticks, and Shake

Meal 5: Low-Carb Meal
>   Recipe: Creamy Cauliflower Soup

Fitness Testing Day

Just like stepping on the scale to get a measure for your current weight, we need to get a measure for your fitness level. Don't worry, this won't take long—only 4 minutes total. However, if you haven't been active for quite some time, you may feel a little soreness tomorrow! At the end of the 21 Days to Extreme Transformation we will test you again, and you will be blown away at the difference! The challenge here is to set a clock for one minute and perform as many repetitions of the following exercises as you can 3—2—1...go!

See Part 4, The Metabolic Movements, for step-by-step instructions on the following exercises. Set a running clock and do as many reps as you can in 1 minute. Record your time in the Daily Tracker to complete the mission!

Push-Ups
Sit-Ups
Squats
Burpees

Day 1: Metabolic Mission: Go the Distance (Stepladder)

Your mission is to start at 3 reps each of the movements below and increase 3 reps every circuit (for example 3, 6, 9, 12, 15, 18...). How many circuits can you do in 12 minutes of these three exercises? Record how far you make it in your tracker!

Kickbacks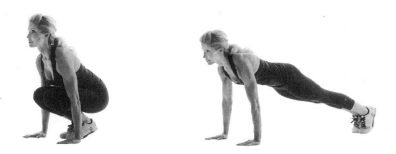

Push-Ups

Back Lunges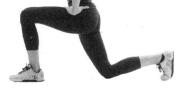

Get ready...3—2—1...go!!

Day 1: Accelerator: 5 minutes (minimum)

Select any activity of your choosing (see page 89 for a list of activities), and keep your heart rate above 120 beats per minute (bpm) the entire time. Prescribed optional interval for maximum results: Mighty Minutes (1:00 low intensity / 1:00 high intensity).

LESSON 1
FIND YOUR *WHAT* AND YOUR *WHY*

Life isn't about finding yourself. Life is about creating yourself.
—George Bernard Shaw

To be successful on any journey, you *must* have a clear-cut picture of where you want to go. This journey is no exception. You *must* know ahead of time what your goal is, and why you want it. This begs the extremely important question: *What* do you want to achieve from Extreme Transformation?

Now is not the time to be vague. We are naturally programmed to give simple and nebulous answers like "I just want to be healthier" or "I want to be fitter." In transformation, these goals are absolutely unacceptable. There is no way to measure them, so you can justify reaching them at any time. We tend to make these unclear goals subconsciously so that we aren't held accountable to any true commitment.

Not this time.

One of the keys to maximizing the impact of the Extreme Transformation is setting SMART goals. Transformation cannot begin until a SMART goal is set. So what is a SMART goal? A goal that is:

1. **Specific**—What you want must be laid out in precise detail. Ask yourself the question, *What exactly will I achieve?* The next few components will help you dial in the specificity of your goal.

2. **Measurable**—What you will achieve must be able to be measured to verify whether it was achieved or not. It must be quantifiable! Pounds lost, inches lost, medical numbers, clothing sizes, and performance times are all measurable and acceptable for your goal! In addition, because your goal is measurable, you can regularly measure your progress to see if you are on track. Numbers don't lie, and they can keep you moving in the right direction or help you refocus your efforts.

3. **Attainable**—A successful goal must be attainable—not too difficult or idealistic, or you're setting yourself up for failure from Day 1. Yes, you could say your goal is to exercise five days a week for 30 minutes, but let's be honest: Sometimes life gets in the way and the best plans go out the window. What

happens then? You break a commitment and you feel like a failure. You need to make your goal attainable—one you know that you can keep every single day—and you'll be well on your way to success. You'll love those daily feelings of accomplishment so much that you might even do more than you've promised yourself you'd do (like exercising more than five minutes a day)!

4. **Relevant**—A SMART goal must be important enough to you that you'll want to make the necessary sacrifices to achieve it. It must be a major priority in your life, to the point at which it creates a sense of urgency in your life.

5. **Time-Sensitive**—A SMART goal must have a time limit so you won't get sidetracked and not accomplish it. Placing a time limit on your goal creates a sense of urgency that will make it a priority. There must be a specific window of time in which the goal is achieved. Eventually, sometime, or next year will never happen. Your goal will not be complete until you put a hard date on it.

Call to Action: Declaring Your Dream

It's time to create your first SMART goal. Today you are going to create a goal for the transformation journey with us. For example: *I will lose 20 pounds in 60 days*. One final note before you declare your SMART goal: Our choice of words is extremely important here. We must leave no wiggle room for our goals to escape us. We *never* use the wording *I want to* or *I'll try*—that type of phrasing plants the seed of avoidance and gives you an out. In declaring your goal, use the words *I will*. This transformation is the real deal, and you *will* be held to your word.

It is time now for you. Take some time to think about it, then in the space below write it down and declare your goal. It must start with *I will* and finish with a specific date by which it will be completed. Maybe your goal with us is to lose a certain number of pounds; maybe it's something else. You are the artist…paint your picture below, and tell us what you *will* achieve:

_____

_____

_____

_____

Find Your Why

Nice work creating such a powerful SMART goal! It isn't easy to make such a solid commitment, but those who have the courage to take these steps have what it takes to change forever. Now that we have identified where we want to go with your SMART goal, we're going to help you discover something just as important: your why. This is the motivating force that is going to keep you on track the whole way.

So why is this goal important to you? Why do you want to lose weight? Why do you want to transform? *Defining your why* is the driving force of your journey and is something that should not be taken lightly.

Pay close attention: Our why is our motivation!

Ever lose your motivation? Exactly. That's why we need to know our why, and keep it in front of us at all times. It is a main key to long-term success on this journey!

The decision to begin this journey of transformation occurs for many reasons, for many different kinds of people. Many decisions to lose weight are triggered by huge life events, sometimes even traumatic events. For some people it's a health scare—a report that delivers a diagnosis such as diabetes, the precursors of heart disease, or high blood pressure. Others are confronted by a realization that their lives are just not working anymore—that life as they know it is painful, and they desire more. Some choose to make changes because of a sudden loss or trauma in their lives, an event so cataclysmic that the desire for deep change feels like survival. Others decide to lose weight for those around them, saying to themselves, "*If I lose weight, I can be a better spouse, parent, or child.*"

Many people reach a rock bottom, a point of realization that their current condition of living is so toxic and unbearable that they can no longer fathom another day in the same way. As Tony Robbins said, "Change happens when the pain of staying the same is greater than the pain of change."

For Mike, his why came in the form of hearing the news from his doctor that his heart was going to fail if he didn't radically change his habits. With an 11-year-old child, he realized that not only did his own life depend upon his becoming healthy, but his son's did as well.

For David, it was the moment walking down the street when he saw his reflection in a window and said to himself, "*Who's that fat guy?*" before he realized that he wasn't the fit young man he used to be. He wanted to be fit and healthy again.

For Merhbod, finding his why occurred when his girlfriend presented him with a tape recording of him sleeping. The tape revealed that his sleep apnea had become so bad that every few minutes he would stop breathing for 45 to 60 seconds. Mehrbod was shocked and decided at that moment that he had to change before he might literally stop breathing and die in his sleep.

For Josh, transformation began after his father died. The loss devastated him, but it brought him a crystal-clear moment when he realized that he was not living the life his father would want for him. "This was not my life," Josh remembers saying to himself. "No one knew how unhappy I was. I was closed off from everyone. But deep down I wanted more from life, and I deserved more from life. So I went out and took it because I knew that life wasn't going to hand it to me!"

Juliana wanted to walk down the halls of her high school with confidence.

Cassie wanted to look the son she'd put up for adoption in the face without feeling ashamed of herself.

Kenny wanted to feel like the proud U.S. Marine he'd once been.

Cassandra wanted to be the athlete she used to be.

Other people's whys are much less dark and complicated. Your why might simply be that you want to look good at your high school reunion. Or maybe to drop a couple sizes to fit into some smaller jeans. Some people just want to lose the baby weight to feel sexy for their significant other again! As Kristen remembers, "I've been there! After devoting nine months to growing a baby and another year to nursing, multiplied by four babies, I was simply ready to feel strong, powerful, beautiful, and sexy again. I wanted my body to feel like something I controlled for once in 10 years of the pregnancy process…not a body that was controlled by external forces any longer."

Whys don't have to be dramatic, but they do need to come from a place of passion. You've got to want it more than you want anything else and be willing to make this a priority, like you would an emergency or crisis, or you will not have the drive to do what it takes to complete the journey. What do *you* want more from this than anything else? What is your why?

Finding the Clarity of Your Why

Our motivation to change can be boiled down to our two most primal emotions: fear (the force behind you) and love (the force in front of you). The way we see it, either there is something you are running from, or something you are running toward—or a little bit of both! Every why has one or both of these two emotions driving it: one that you are wanting to move *away* from (*fear*), and one that you are wanting to move *toward* (*love*). Which one you choose to focus on is totally up to you.

Fear-based whys tend to be the situations or feelings that we are running away from—bad health, unacceptable appearance, depression and self-loathing, upset/frustration of spouse/family members, fear of death, and so on. These emotions scare us and so we turn to transformation as a way out. Love-based whys are motivating situations or feelings that we actually run toward—that perfect beach body, the ability to run and play with your kids, the possibility of being an athlete, six-pack abs, a spouse who loves and accepts you. When your why is love-based, it's positive, affirming, and ultimately more liberating.

But that's not to discount fear-based whys: Often this is the powerful place many of us start at, and that is okay. The most important point to keep in mind is that you start—even if it is a fear-based why that helps get you to begin your journey of transformation. Eventually, you may likely shift to a love-based why.

Take a look at how some of the common ways people explain their whys to us fall into the two categories, love-based and fear-based:

Fear—"I have too much physical pain and discomfort—I can barely move around anymore."

Love—"I want to be able to move freely without pain."

Fear—"My relationship is getting worse and worse. My partner is going to leave me."

Love—"I want to love myself more, so I can be a better person for my partner—and our relationship can thrive."

Fear—"I don't want to be lonely anymore."

Love—"I want to look better so I can meet others and date with confidence."

You get it. We're either running away from something we don't want, or running toward something we do want. There is no right or wrong here. While we do hope to help you and every person ultimately find a why based on love at some point of their journey, you might not be there yet. The fact of the matter is that you are here and you are reading this book…taking that first step toward a new you!

Call to Action: Declare It!

Looking through the lists above, take a moment to think about your why and ask yourself these two questions:

1. Why is your goal important to you?

_____
_____
_____
_____

2. Is it fear-based or love-based?

_____

Remember: If you don't want to lose motivation, you must memorialize your why. Put it in multiple places you will see every day. These are common places where our participants have placed their whys:

- Bathroom mirror
- Dashboard
- Workplace or desk
- Refrigerator
- Living room
- Cell phone home screen

Do not read any further until you have taken action. Put this book down and immediately memorialize your why. Don't risk losing your motivation ever again. Put it everywhere you can to remind yourself!

Next, share your why with others. If you are still scared of the commitment, try sharing it with one friend. If you are ready to rock, post it online for all of your friends! Better yet, post it on *our* social networks and let our community support you in achieving your why! #extremetransformation

Facebook:
RealHeidiPowell
RealChrisPowell
Twitter:
@RealHeidiPowell
@RealChrisPowell
Instagram:
@RealHeidiPowell
@RealChrisPowell

Reality Check

You will likely forget why you're doing this every now and then. Your pictures will likely lose their impact and you will become desensitized to seeing the same pic in the same place every day. To stay motivated, keep telling others about your goals. Try putting up new pics every week or two. Change their location; do whatever it takes to keep it fresh!

In difficult times, you may try to convince yourself that you don't really want your why, or that it has changed. While it is perfectly okay for your why to shift as you get to know yourself through this process, it isn't okay to tell yourself that you never really wanted your why in the first place... and this is all too easy to do when the going gets tough. Don't lie to yourself. You want it and you know it. It's yours, so go get it!

Heidi Tip

We usually ask our peeps to identify their why and then make a collage that they can place around their home, or even a collage of photos or an avatar for their phone that represents their why. For example, Tanya's why was "I choose to transform so that I never have to be the girl hiding in the back of every picture!" She made a collage of herself standing in the back, hiding, in a handful of pics. If your why has something to do with becoming more active and connected to your family, you might create a collage with some photos of you sitting with your kids and then other pics of a mom (like you!) running, jumping, swimming, or playing in the park or on the beach! The point is to choose images that inspire you!

The Deeper Why

Often what we *think* is our why is just scratching the surface of what we *really* want. We're not saying that your why isn't valid, because whatever comes up for you is real and true. But what we've learned through the years of helping hundreds of people successfully lose excess pounds is that your first why may be just the surface of a much deeper well of understanding. So keep checking in with yourself and be aware that your first why may be a powerful stepping-stone toward a much more important why inside yourself.

As you dig deeper into yourself (and as you do the 21 steps), you very well may (and *should*!) realize that your why is actually deeper than you initially thought. As Mark explains, "I wanted more than anything to find the love of my life, and I know I couldn't do that at 650 pounds. I wanted the girl of my dreams!"

But what Mark didn't realize at the time was that his why was so much deeper than just wanting to find a wife. As he followed his own journey of transformation—as he continually focused on improving himself (and being open, honest, and vulnerable)—he "peeled back those layers" of protection that had masked his true self. How did he finally get to his deeper why? He kept asking himself why and listened to his own answers:

"Well, why do I want the girl of my dreams so bad? Because that would make me happy, whole, and complete. I've never had that before."

"Why do I need someone else to make me feel happy, whole, and complete? Because I can't seem to find happiness on my own…I am not happy."

"Why and how would another human being fill this void then?"

Well, that was the critical question that led to Mark's true why.

For Mark, his deeply rooted answer boiled down to simply trying to fill the basic human need to be loved and accepted. And while this *need* doesn't have to come from another, he felt a wife would give him the love and acceptance he craved.

After time working his inner steps, Mark ultimately realized that when he started to love and accept himself by keeping his promises and finding integrity, he was able to rely much less on validation, love, and acceptance from others and rely much more on himself—all the love and acceptance he needed was within him!

DAY 2

Day 2: High-Carb Day

Meal 1: Breakfast
Recipe: Scrambled Eggs and Hash

Meal 2: High-Carb Meal
Recipe: Lemon Poppy Seed Protein Bites

Meal 3: High-Carb Meal
Recipe: Chicken Fajita Bowl

Meal 4: High-Carb Meal
Recipe: Homemade Tortilla Chips with Tomato Salsa

Meal 5: Low-Carb Meal
Recipe: Shrimp and Chicken Stir-Fry

Day 2: Metabolic Mission: The Whole 9 (RFT)

Set a running clock and do 9 rounds as fast as you can of the following circuit. Record your time in the tracker to complete the mission!

Air Squats: 9 reps
Hollow Rocks: 9 reps
Push-Ups: 9 reps

Day 2: Accelerator: 5 minutes (minimum)

Select any activity of your choosing, and keep your heart rate above 120 beats per minute (bpm) the entire time. Prescribed optional interval for maximum results: Dirty Two-Thirties (2:30 low intensity / 2:30 high intensity)

LESSON 2
DISCOVER THE TRUE PATH TO TRANSFORMATION

The only journey is the one within.

—Rainer Maria Rilke

Do a Google search for "weight loss" and within seconds you will see hundreds (if not thousands) of different diets, programs, and plans that promise a set of guidelines to help you lose weight. Guess what? *Most* of them work. So with widespread access for much of the world to this free information, why isn't everyone lean and healthy? They all tout being the "path" to your weight loss goals. So why do 9 out of 10 people fail on these diets? Why haven't we found the universal answer to weight loss?

Because we're looking in the wrong place.

There is only *one* true path to what you really want.

We have been blinded by so much confusion everywhere, with every weight loss program pitching that they have "the answer" to your problems with new diets and exercises, that we've never thought to look where the path *really* is—and what lifelong success is really all about—the journey within. Inside all of us is the secret path to our true selves, which coincides with being *at* our ideal weight. It already exists. It has been there all along. We are intrinsically programmed to follow it, but we must see the journey for what it really is...and never underestimate its power.

This path has all the answers—why you've failed in the past, why you lost belief in yourself, why you feel the way you do right now, and why you are struggling with those extra pounds. This path will lead to your goal weight and body, but ultimately it will lead you to loving and appreciating yourself. It will lead you to joy, confidence, and esteem greater than you can imagine. It's ready and waiting for you to explore it.

What we are talking about is the path of *integrity.*

Please pay close attention. When you understand the path of integrity and follow it, your whole life changes. Immediately. *This* is the secret we have used with all of our transformations over the years—and every single one will tell you that it changed their lives forever.

Before we dive in deep, let's define it.

What is integrity?

Integrity is...

Doing what you say you are going to do, when you say you are going to do it.

We are going to say something that may upset you here. We are going to be so bold as to say that you likely have *not* had integrity with yourself. You're probably reading this thinking, "Well, screw you guys. I have integrity. Anytime I tell someone I'm going to do something, darn it, I do it!"

We're sure you probably do have integrity with *other* people. Heck, if you make a commitment to someone, you've got to follow through, right? Well, try this scenario: What if you made a promise to the most important person in the world. Would you do it? Before you answer, think long and hard about it. Because there *is* one person in this world who has the greatest power to impact your life and your *quality* of life—you.

Let's try something—if you've been following the path of integrity with yourself, then how many times have you said, "The diet starts Monday"? or, "I'm going to set my clock an hour early to exercise tomorrow morning." How about, "2010—this is my year!" How about 2011? 2012? 2013? 2014? 2015?

Get the point? If you had followed the path of integrity, you would have only made the promise *once*. Right now, you'd be at your goal.

You see, we spend so much time making and breaking promises to ourselves, we reach the point that eventually when we make yet *another* promise to lose the weight, we don't believe ourselves anymore…it's just going to be another failed attempt…because we don't believe *in* ourselves anymore.

We're sure that for each of these failed attempts, there are a million reasons why it didn't work. However, understand this: Your integrity does not know excuses. You either do it, or you don't.

Engrain this truth in your mind, and it will change your life forever:

When you say you are going to do something…do it. Our promises are one of the single most powerful forces in existence. In order to make any progress in life, in order to transform ourselves, we must make promises to ourselves and keep them. However, what most of us don't realize is that *every time* we make a promise to ourselves, we are putting our most valuable asset on the line—our dignity. Our dignity is our confidence, our esteem, our self-love, our ability to believe in ourselves. If we keep the promise, our dignity grows even more. If we don't, the broken promise can trigger a catastrophic backslide. (More to come in Lesson 3!)

Call to Action: The Feeling of Integrity

When we complete a commitment, or keep a promise, we are left with a feeling of being whole, complete, fulfilled, and satisfied.

1. List three times you've followed through with what you said you were going to do—both for yourself and for others.

_____
_____
_____
_____

_____
_____

2. How did you feel about yourself when you did it?

_____
_____
_____

Now…take that feeling and amplify it by 1,000. When you start keeping your promises to yourself, it's kind of like that... but even better. ☺

Integrity is not only the essence of once again feeling whole and loving yourself, but also the root of human change. Each time you honor your word, not just to others, but most important to yourself, you take control of your destiny and put yourself in the driver's seat of your own life. Each time you make and keep a promise to yourself, you show yourself that you have control over what you say and do.

When you follow through and do something that you said you were going to do, you become more dependable and solid to yourself. The result? You not only grow your integrity but also achieve a greater level of dignity—the quality of being worthy of honor or respect. Yes—your integrity grows your dignity. And the reward for building a life based on integrity is dignity—the love, respect, and esteem of yourself.

From this moment on, you must realize that while the nutrition of the Extreme Cycle and the power of Metabolic Missions and Accelerators will help you lose weight quickly and effectively, they are *not* the answer to your transformation. Your integrity is. Your ability to honor your word to yourself. When you do what you say you are going to do—when you say you are going to do it—you will execute the Extreme Cycle, Metabolic Missions, and Accelerators beautifully, leading to extraordinary results. Your focus should now and forever be first and foremost on keeping your promises to yourself. When that happens, everything else falls into place. Are you starting to understand it now?

When our people stand on stage at the end of their yearlong journey, with their chest out and their chin high, they no longer care about the number on the scale. (It was simply a SMART goal that they achieved—by doing what they said they were going to do, when they said they were going to do it.) They look and feel that way because they *love* themselves. They know what the journey is *really* about. For example, if they made a commitment to do 30 minutes on a treadmill, and one of us pulled them off at 29 minutes, they would throw a punch at us. They would literally fight us to complete that last minute. Why? Will one minute on a treadmill make *any* difference in their weight loss? Nope. But they know what is on the line—their dignity—and nothing is worth jeopardizing that. If they broke their promise, it could trigger a devastating backslide of more broken promises. They know where the true value is—not in the exercise, not in the diet, but in themselves and their promises.

They became promise keepers, and it led them to the ultimate reward. And oh yeah, because of it they lost a lot of weight, too. ☺

Georgeanna recalls, "In the beginning, I really needed Chris and Heidi and the rest of the team to believe in me. It took me making and keeping my own promises to believe that I really could do it. I remember one day Chris asked me, 'Georgeanna, why is it that you can make and keep all sorts of promises to other people, but you can't keep them for yourself?'—a lightbulb went on and I just understood why it was so important for me to put myself first. That's how I began to really believe in myself."

Each day you follow this path, you walk toward a profound sense of self-love. And when you reach this place, it's not an end of a journey but rather an opening to a vast and endless source of vitality, meaning, fulfillment, and peace. This is where you will live. And this is what transformation is all about.

Take a look at the stereogram image below. This captures the essence of transformation so beautifully. Before you shift your focus, all you see is a chaotic mess of dumbbells and food. Basically, it is the confusing mess of every single diet and exercise program out there for weight loss. But once you shift your focus, the 3-D path of true transformation—and lifelong weight loss—becomes clear.

Transformation path viewing tips:

1. With your eyes about 18 to 24 inches from the image, choose a spot in the center of it and stare directly at it.
2. Continue to stare at the image and let your eyes relax. Focus your eyes as if you are trying to look through the image at something behind it.
3. Your eyes may go slightly out of focus—this is okay.
4. After a short period of time, you may start to see some depth appear on the image. If this is the case, then you are very close. Hold your eyes on the same spot and continue to let the hidden image move toward you.
5. If you do it properly, you will now start to see the hidden image.
6. If you still can't see the image, keep trying. There is a hidden image or 3-D element in this image. Don't give up!

The Hidden Path Stereogram

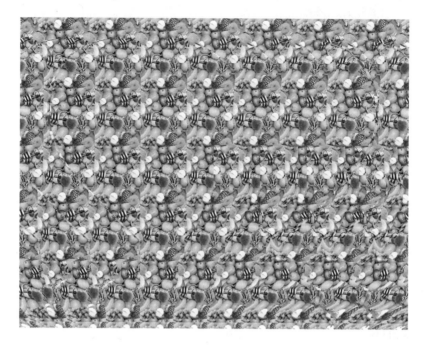

She was looking outside herself for answers, instead of inside. And when she changed her focus to her integrity, to keeping her promises, she never looked back.

The stereogram image represents the path of integrity that lies inside each one of us. Each step up represents a promise you make and keep. These steps combine and form your goals—daily goals, weekly goals, monthly and yearly goals. Your promise-filled life is an ever-rising stairway to your best self.

As you can see the stereogram is built upon a stairway of such promises; they build on one another and head in only one direction—up, toward the top. What's at the top of this staircase? Dignity. Esteem. Confidence. Self-love. And once you have that, you have everything. The world is your oyster...you can conquer and achieve anything.

Jacqui describes her Extreme Transformation and what it felt like when she discovered her why, and connected to her inner path to integrity and self-love. "We all can get stuck in our lives, but I feel so lucky. I didn't believe I could change or had the power to change. I tried and failed time and again. This mind-set reinforced that I was not good enough, so I stayed in that cycle of broken promises and failure. I believed the lies about myself. But Chris and Heidi believed in me—for me. They showed me the true path to transformation, and it finally all made sense. I realized it was a battle with my mind and my heart, not my body."

Call to Action

The absolute essence of the shift in mind-set that needs to happen throughout your transformation journey requires that you get to the realization that the power to change is within you. So if you are ready to transform, read this out loud and own it:

"I know the hidden path to transformation lies in my integrity. I understand the extreme value of my promises and their power over my results and the way I feel about myself. From this moment on, I am a promise keeper to myself."

Reality Check

On the way, it is easy to forget that transformation is about integrity, and get wrapped back up in the numbers game. You'll get desperate to turn numbers on the scale and start looking for other fad diets and quick fixes to get the number you want to see. At this point, your focus will shift back to the chaos of the thousands of diet and exercise programs out there.

Keep this book close. Remember, it is your guide. Read through the lessons over and over again. And remember, your path is within you.

DAY 3

Day 3: High-Carb Day

Meal 1: Breakfast
    Recipe: No-Bake Oats

Meal 2: High-Carb Meal
    Recipe: Honey Dijon Chicken Snack Wrap

Meal 3: High-Carb Meal
    Recipe: Butternut Squash Chili

Meal 4: High-Carb Meal
    Recipe: Apple and Dip

Meal 5: Low-Carb Meal
    Recipe: Cheesy Chicken and String Beans

Day 3: Metabolic Mission: Burpee Love (Chipper)

Set a running clock and see how long it takes to complete the mission. Record your time in your Daily Tracker! Ready? 3—2—1...go!

60 Burpees

Day 3: Accelerator: 5 minutes (minimum)

Select any activity of your choosing, and keep your heart rate above 120 beats per minute (bpm) the entire time. Prescribed optional interval for maximum results: Thrilling Thirties (:30 low intensity / :30 high intensity)

LESSON 3
KEEP YOUR PROMISES

The journey of 1,000 miles begins with a single step.

—Lao Tzu

To put things into perspective: Every diet and exercise program (including this one) involves a series of promises. To make it clear for you, we have identified the three most powerful, universal promises of Extreme Transformation:

1. Eat according to the Extreme Cycle high- and low-carb days, with portions, recipes, and acceptable foods.
2. Do a Metabolic Mission five days per week.
3. Do an Accelerator six days per week.

Keeping these promises will lead to significant weight loss. If you are able to take on all of these promises all at once, that's fantastic. You will achieve your goals in record time! However, it's time for a reality check. If you cannot keep all of these promises, you *must* only commit to the ones you know you *can* do. Just as kept promises are the powerful steps toward a lean and fit body, loving yourself, and believing in yourself, broken promises are the devastating reciprocate. A single, small broken promise can trigger a catastrophic backslide of weight gain, crushed esteem, and lost belief in ourselves.

Silent Promises

For the first few attempts at weight loss, most of us have told others our intentions and promises. Failure after failure, we lose more and more belief in ourselves, and usually feel ashamed when others question our resolve. When we lose belief in ourselves, we begin to do something dangerous—we make silent promises. Heaven forbid you commit to starting a program in front of your family, friends, or co-workers, right? Because come Thursday and you are housing a whole stuffed crust pizza in the break room, you're going to have some explaining to do, right? When we are not ready to truly commit, or don't believe in our ability to succeed, we make *silent promises* to ourselves. We whisper to ourselves that "the diet starts Monday." Our ego avoids declaring them in front of others in case we do fall—so that it avoids the shame of looking bad and weak in front of others, and possibly losing connection with them. The voice in our head tells us that if nobody heard the promise, then we can just sweep it under the rug when we break it—no harm done, right? Wrong. More harm done than had you never made the promise in the first place. Promises are promises, silent or not! You don't realize it, but you gambled with your dignity again...and you lost.

So here's where it gets nasty—when you break a promise, you don't just go back to square one. You drop twice as far. Promise after promise broken leads to more and more darkness, despair, and self-hatred. If many of you are wondering how and why you found yourself in such a dark place, *this is the answer.* You've been playing with fire all along and you never even knew it. When we meet our people for the first time, we don't see hundreds of pounds of extra weight—we see hundreds of pounds of broken promises.

Promises should never be silent. They should be said out loud. And they should be SMART! Just like your goals, you need to keep your promises simple and smart (you may want to revisit the SMART goals you declared in Lesson 1). You also want to declare them—to yourself and to others.

Keep in mind that every time you failed at weight loss in the past can be traced back to a single moment when you broke your integrity. Every backslide begins the moment you *don't* do what you said you were going to do. It doesn't matter the circumstances. Go back in your past and think about it...

Seriously...think about it.

On the course of *every* program you've followed in the past, the backslide began with one slip—one broken promise.

Not this time.

Now that you know the power of our promises and how they can cut both ways, the only promises you should ever make from this moment on are the ones that you *know* you can keep. The journey to loving yourself is done one simple promise at a time.

The beauty of the path to your true self is simple: It is uncovered as soon as you make a single promise to yourself and fulfill that promise. The bricks-and-mortar of your integrity will rise every time you keep that promise. Dignity and self-love are both by-products of integrity. Although they may seem minuscule, these small promises are the foundation to profound change.

"Starting now, I will eat breakfast every day."

"From now on, I'm going to drink flavored water instead of soda."

"I will ride the stationary bike for five minutes every morning."

When you make such simple promises to yourself and you keep them day after day, you begin to grow your trust in yourself that you can actually *keep* that promise. You begin to...wait for it...

Believe in yourself.

Maybe even for the first time. But over time, once you believe and trust yourself to keep a promise, you begin to wonder what else you can do. So you make another small promise—and keep it. It is a wonderful upward climb of integrity and curiosity! You feel love for yourself, you have dignity, and you build what we call "integrity momentum."

The more you keep your promises, the more you don't want to break the streak! Integrity momentum is like a freight train. It starts out slow, but once it gets moving you can't stop it. This is exactly what we do with the participants on the show. They build up so much integrity momentum, you can't stop them!

Now let's put this into weight loss perspective. When you focus on fulfilling your promises based on diet and exercise, weight loss happens! You keep the promise, goals are achieved. Period.

So how do you get started? In our second book, we offered a list of 101 Power Promises—these are a collection of effective, single promises that you can use to set the foundation and take the first step in your transformation journey. We took those 101 promises and simplified them down to the most vital 20 promises for you to choose from. For your Power Promise, you can select one of these provided, or you can choose your own!

Heather was a chronic sumo dieter—she was never hungry in the morning, so she skipped breakfast, went to work, never ate a thing until late lunch. By that time she was so hungry she could (and would) eat anything. She ended up stuffing her face for late lunch and then again when she came home from work. She was so hungry late in the day she would eat until she went to bed. Heather began her transformation journey by Power Promising that she would wake up half an hour earlier in the morning so she had time for breakfast. That was her first promise to herself and by keeping it, she learned something hugely important: She was able to show up for herself each day. We put no calorie limits on breakfast, and she could choose anything—because the promise was just to eat breakfast. It became a victory each morning to start her day. The feeling was contagious, and it spread to other aspects of her life. After a couple weeks of keeping this Power Promise, she began to grow more and more confident in her ability to actually do it...like really, truly stick to it!

Once she was so confident she could keep her Power Promise, it was time to make her second promise. Her second promise to herself? She ate every three hours. At first, this didn't feel comfortable—she felt like she was eating too much. But the result was surprising. "I felt no need to overeat; I never felt hungry. Oddly enough, the scale started going down. I simply felt great!" One year and a few more promises later, and Heather is now 140 pounds lighter and a self-proclaimed promise keeper.

Promises to ourselves are the mini steps that lead to our goals. John's first promise to himself was to stop eating at drive-thrus. As a trucker, he is on the road all the time. He eats in his truck, sleeps in his truck, and for all intents and purposes lives in his truck. Making this promise to himself meant that John had to stop, park, and move to eat. He had to get out of his truck and walk into a diner or other low-key restaurant that served non-processed foods. This required time, patience, and energy. But John believed that he could. He believed that he had the power to follow through on this one initial promise. And each day he fulfilled this promise, he began to feel differently about himself. Instead of that "inside me" voice that said he was lazy and fat, he began to hear another voice: "*You're doing great, boy—keep it up!*" He was becoming his own coach. As the days passed, it got easier and easier to avoid the drive-thru. In addition, because walking into a restaurant was a conscious decision based upon his new commitment, he was more aware of the foods he was eating and naturally chose to make healthier choices. Even when he was short on time, he had gone so long without giving in to temptation that to him, it wasn't even an option anymore. At the end of two months, he not only had lost thirty-six pounds, he felt better, stronger, and more confident.

Defining Your Power Promises

Being on your path, continuing to make promises to yourself and keeping them, requires focus and energy. It asks you to make one promise at a time and fulfill it, so you can build the scaffolding of your path to self-love. That's the essence of growing integrity and, ultimately, dignity. But once your path reveals itself, you are free to choose your destiny. Now you know, and you can never unlearn it!

You may have thought that eating right and exercising are the foundation of long-term weight loss. But now you know that that's not the case. As so many of our clients will tell you, the reason they were able to drop 10 or 20 sizes or shed 50 to 200 pounds was because they changed their life one promise at a time.

The key to transformation—we tell them again and again—is this: The more you build your integrity, the more dignity you grow. Every time you make a promise to yourself, your self-esteem, the very basis of your integrity, is on the line.

So how do you get started? Of course you can name any promise you want, but we want to give you some direction on how to define your promises and how these lead to and support your goals (which you will declare in the next step). Your Power Promises can fall into multiple categories, like: food promises, body promises, and mind promises. We have identified **20 Daily Power Promises** to jump-start you.

A Power Promise is something that is committed to daily.

1. I will eat breakfast within 30 minutes of waking up.
2. I will reduce drinking alcohol to one day a week or not at all.
3. I will drink an extra quart of water every day.
4. I will drink a cup of water before each meal.
5. I will stop drinking soda.
6. I will eat five meals a day.
7. I will eat protein first at every meal.

8. I will not eat my kids' food.
9. I will not eat after my fifth meal.
10. I will not eat in the car.
11. I will not eat fast food.
12. I will not add salt to my food.
13. I will eat veggies of at least two different colors every day.
14. I will take a brisk walk every morning or lunch break every day.
15. I will exercise for at least five minutes every day.
16. I will not watch TV unless I do exercises during the commercial breaks.
17. I will set my alarm 30 minutes early every morning to make time for my exercise.
18. I will track my food every day.
19. I will not eat when watching TV or using the computer.
20. I will pay attention to my hunger and only eat when I'm physically hungry.

Call to Action

Keep in mind that these Power Promises are suggestions. But understand the power of the promise you choose, and that your integrity and dignity (and ultimately your success) are on the line here. You can adapt these promises, replace them, and add to them. It's all up to you. What's important is that you declare a promise that you can repeat each day, stick to it, and acknowledge to yourself that you did so. This conscious awareness of your accomplishments is an important part of your motivation and growing belief in yourself.

If you read between the lines of the 20 Daily Power Promises, you might notice the outlines of the healthy lifestyle that we are introducing. (Feel free to go back and check on the exact instructions for the Extreme Cycle in chapter 2.) But for now, if you're not ready to take on the whole Extreme Cycle, Metabolic Missions, and Accelerators just use *one* of these Power Promises to get you started on the right foot. Make one promise to yourself each day and keep it. Continue to make that daily commitment. When that promise becomes almost automatic, then build another promise on top of it. As you fulfill promise after promise, you will see and feel your body and mind changing. The resulting feeling of accomplishment and contentment is indescribable. You will experience a whole new sense of control over your life that you've never felt before.

So how do you make this happen?

Here's a great strategy that has worked for our clients:

1. Write down your Power Promise and post it in at least three places where you will see it often—your bathroom mirror, laptop screen, smartphone, workplace, or even your refrigerator.

2. Declare your promise to someone and ask for that person's support. In addition, send an email, a text, a post on Facebook—any form of communication or announcement that works for you. See our FB page to give you more suggestions on how to boost your motivation and get the most from your Transformation Team!

3. Prepare what you need to keep this commitment to yourself. For instance, if your Power Promise is to walk instead of drive, what does that entail? Do you have to leave for work earlier? Do you need to take a different kind of bag to work—a backpack to hold your meals, instead of a shoulder bag that will weigh you down? Think ahead and make adjustments as necessary to ensure you can keep your promise.

By the end of a week, go through these three steps and see how you feel. If you were able to keep that promise for one day or seven, acknowledge your victory!

Reality Check

You will likely find yourself tempted to take on multiple promises again. If you can keep them, more power to you! Enjoy your rapid results! However, if you can't keep all of the promises, know that the consequences are disastrous. If you need to, shrink your list of promises so that you are committed to only the ones that you *know* you can keep.

Heads up: You are likely going to break your Power Promise sometime along the journey. See Lesson 16: Fall Without Failing for the formula to get back on your feet. With this formula, you can never fail!

DAY 4

Day 4: High-Carb Day

Meal 1: Breakfast
    Recipe: Egg and Cheddar Sandwich

Meal 2: High-Carb Meal
    Recipe: Spiced Banana Shake

Meal 3: High-Carb Meal
    Recipe: BBQ Baked Sweet Potato, Loaded with Grilled Chicken, Corn, and Black Beans

Meal 4: High-Carb Meal
    Recipe: Triple Berry Treat

Meal 5: Low-Carb Meal
    Recipe: Zucchini and Turkey "Lasagna Roll-Ups"

Day 4: Metabolic Mission: Phoenix Rising (AMRAP)

Set a running clock and perform as many rounds of the following circuit as you can in 15 minutes. Record your rounds in your Daily Tracker!

5 Push-Ups
10 Sit-Ups
15 Squats

Day 4: Accelerator: 5 minutes (minimum)

Select any activity of your choosing, and keep your heart rate above 120 beats per minute (bpm) the entire time. Prescribed optional interval for maximum results: Tenacious Twos (2:00 low intensity / 2:00 high intensity)

LESSON 4
PREPARE FOR SUCCESS

By failing to prepare, you are preparing to fail.

—Benjamin Franklin

Success doesn't just happen. You must create it. Now that you understand and "see" the true path to transformation, it's time to get down to the nitty-gritty. With SMART goals set, your why in place, and the arsenal of all your other empowering steps under your belt, this lesson is simple, practical, and super critical to your ultimate success!

Proper nutrition will account for the majority of your weight loss success. Because of this, we have designed 21 days of delicious recipes for you. But let's get real here: Some recipes you will love, and some you may not. We designed these 21 days for you to try all kinds of different food combinations and possibilities for two reasons:

1. To help you find the recipes that you love and stick with them.
2. To give you some awesome ideas to get creative with your own food combinations and recipes.

If you love the recipes and have the time to create them, then use them to cycle away to your goal weight! But if you are limited on time or have specific tastes when it comes to your food, this lesson is for you.

Create Your Own Meals

If you have specific tastes, or if you want to get creative with your own Extreme Cycle meal combinations, the formula is simple:

1. Create your daily menus by selecting your favorite foods (Protein, Carbs, Fats, and Veggies) from the Acceptable Foods list.
2. Follow the prescribed Extreme Cycle meal combinations (High-Carb Day, Low-Carb Day, etc.).
3. Use the 100-calorie portion reference chart (see Appendix D) to determine your portions for each meal:

	Breakfast	High-Carb Meal	Low-Carb Meal
MEN			
Protein	200 calories	150 calories	200 calories
Carbs	150 calories	250 calories	<30 calories
Fats	150 calories	<30 calories	150 calories
WOMEN			
Protein	150 calories	100 calories	150 calories
Carbs	100 calories	200 calories	<30 calories
Fats	100 calories	<30 calories	100 calories

It's that simple. Follow these guidelines for your own custom meals, and Cycle away to a new you.

Whether you follow our recipes or make your own meal combinations, here's the unfortunate catch: If you don't have the right food with you, the usual options are fast food, convenience stores, and vending machines—none of which will likely lead you to your goal. If you want results, you'll need to establish consistency. To make a change in your body, you need to give your body repetition and time. The key to this consistency? Preparing your meals in advance. When you prepare your meals in advance, you guarantee days of nutrition consistency. Day after day, the pounds will be released. Week after week, your clothes will start falling off you and you'll start seeing muscle definition you've never seen before. Month after month, jaws will drop when your family and friends see you! Want this kind of guaranteed success? Meal prep!

Shop, Prep, Store, and Pack

Why is it that nearly everyone who loses a significant amount of weight swears by meal prep? Why is it that all the fittest people in the world meal prep? Why is it that all the people who have lost weight, and *kept* it off for years, preach about meal prep?

Because meal prep works. Because meal prep is the most powerful way to ensure nutrition consistency for the fastest results. Because meal prep is the least expensive and most convenient way to Extreme Cycle and find success on your journey of transformation.

Yes, meal prep takes an hour or two out of your week, but think about it: If you dedicate an hour to preparing your meals in advance, you gain seven days of nutrition success! That is priceless, not to mention the hours of time you will save not having to prepare meals every three hours!

So How Do You Shop?

1. Don't go shopping when you are hungry.
2. Purchase a week of food at a time. Use the shopping lists we provide for the weekly recipes or create your own grocery list.
3. When shopping, stay along the perimeter of the store for most of your groceries, and only go down the aisles that have foods and flavors from the list!

Your Good Food Grocery List

We've organized the grocery lists by food group so that you get accustomed to thinking about all that you eat as either a protein, carbohydrate, vegetable, fat, drink, or flavoring. When you get used to these food groups, making good choices gets easier, and creating delicious dishes is simple! See Appendix B for detailed meal prep instructions for the Extreme Cycle recipes in this book.

How Do You Meal Prep?

Meal prep always seems like a daunting task until you do it—and realize how easy and convenient it really is!

1. Decide which day you are going to shop and meal prep. We usually prep on Sunday. We suggest you prep your foods on your weigh-in/Reset day, or midweek if necessary.
2. Bake, grill, barbecue, and boil all meats and eggs. Flavor using seasonings you choose or sauces from the recipes.
3. Peel, chop, cut, and shred all veggies.
4. Steam, bake, or boil all starches and flavor however you choose.
5. Next, when you're done cooking, allow the dishes to cool, and then portion them out into containers to refrigerate or freeze. Refrigerate foods for meals needed in the next three or four days. Freeze foods for meals after that. And remember to label your containers with the date.
6. Get a cooler, and pack your food for each day to carry with you!

A major component to long-term meal prep is making it easy and convenient. These tools require a onetime purchase, but they will set you up for lifelong success!

- Set of pots and pans
- Set of cutlery
- Blender
- Rice cooker/steamer
- Tabletop grill
- Toaster oven
- Crock-Pot

Reality Check

The reality is that you are going to find yourself in a bind every now and then when you didn't prep when you should have. For those times, you have to make good choices.

If you're in a convenience store, choose nuts, fruit, or a low-sugar protein bar.

If you're in a restaurant, ask your server if they can adapt a dish so that it's clean.

Keep nuts, protein bars, and other healthy snacks in your car or at your desk. If you are on the go or short on time, the following foods require little to no preparation, so they can be ready to go anywhere and anytime. They're also great when traveling—just swing by a grocery store as soon as you reach your destination and stock up!

Proteins

Powdered proteins
Cottage cheese
Plain Greek yogurt
Canned meats
Turkey, chicken, or roast beef deli meat

Carbohydrates

Fruit
Low-fat bran cereals and low-fat granola
Multigrain breads
Beans/lentils
Microwave-ready yams and potatoes

Vegetables

Mixed salads
Frozen veggies in ready-to-microwave
  bags

Fats

String and sliced cheese
Peanut butter and almond butter
Pecans, almonds, and walnuts
Avocado
Salad dressing

DAY 5

Day 5: Low-Carb Day

Meal 1: Breakfast

    Recipe: Green Machine Pancakes

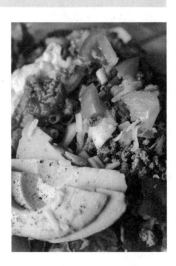

Meal 2: Low-Carb Meal

    Recipe: Stuffed Avocado

Meal 3: Low-Carb Meal

    Recipe: Citrus Salmon Slaw

Meal 4: Low-Carb Meal

    Recipe: Greek Yogurt Parfait with Nuts

Meal 5: Low-Carb Meal

    Recipe: Taco Salad

Day 5: Metabolic Mission: A Lotta Tabata (Tabata)

For each exercise, do as many reps as you can in 20 seconds. Rest for 10 seconds, then do as many reps as you can in 20 seconds again. Repeat for 8 total rounds (for a total of 4 minutes) per exercise. The lowest number of reps you get in any round is your score. You'll get one score per exercise. Add up all three scores, and record it in your Daily Tracker!

Air Squats (lowest reps per round)
Sit-Ups
Push-Ups (lowest reps per round)
Accelerator

Day 5: Accelerator: 5 minutes (minimum)

Select any activity of your choosing, and keep your heart rate above 120 beats per minute (bpm) the entire time. Prescribed optional interval for maximum results: Nasty Nineties (:90 low intensity / :90 high intensity)

LESSON 5
RALLY YOUR TEAM

No man is an island, entire of itself; every man is a piece of the continent.

—John Donne

Team. Support. Comrades. Unity. Something powerful happens when humans come together and cooperate toward a shared vision. They don't become twice as strong; they become exponentially stronger. You might have figured out by now that making this transformation journey alone is a daunting task, and those who have succeeded have done so because they consciously and carefully created a powerful team of supporters. This is not a solo journey: Your path to transformation *requires* interaction with others.

This is where your Transformation Team comes in. Who is this team? They are the people you declare your goals and commitments to. They are the people who hold you accountable. They are the ones who encourage you to keep your promises to yourself—even when you don't want to. They are the ones you lean on when you need to confess and unload emotional baggage. They are your trusted support network. These are people who notice you, care about you, and genuinely support your transformation.

Now, here's the catch: It may or may not be who you think it is. It might be your family and friends. It might be some of your colleagues at work. Or it might be people you don't even know yet.

Your Transformation Team can be anyone from whom you receive love and support.

Bob's Transformation Team is his church. As a devout Christian, Bob relies on his faith to fuel his commitment and keep himself feeling supported and loved. "I have to live authentically," Bob explains. "And for me that means serving others as a way to stay close to my higher power."

Jami formed her own Transformation Team. As she explains, "I started a group called BIG. It's a body image group. As a coach and mentor, I want to support other girls and women around developing a healthy, realistic body image.

Bruce's Transformation Team is—guess who? Us! He not only stays in close contact with us but also "pays it forward," as a mentor to other people who are struggling to lose weight. In turn, these "newbies" have also become Bruce's Transformation Team.

A team member might be a member of your family, church, other support groups, or maybe even people you have met online! We have hundreds of thousands of people on the journey who reach out to us and stay connected through our website, our blog, and our social networks. We invite you to "use us" as your support team. In fact, many of our peeps have connected with one another, creating ever-growing support networks among themselves. Who better to have on your team than someone who understands what the journey is all about?

Yes—these best friends in the world are waiting to meet you! They are friendly, unconditionally supportive, and want you to be healthy and happy!

Reality Check

This may come as a shock, but it is possible that your closest family and friends may not be your biggest supporters. Or maybe they are? When creating your Transformation Team, it is important not to set high expectations of your loved ones, because it can often lead to disappointment. Understand that your goals may not resonate with their goals and aspirations. Your desire to change may threaten them and their lifestyle. It is not uncommon for spouses to be terrified of being abandoned, and best friends afraid of losing their "drinking buddy" or "drive-thru pal." Granted, your wife, brother, or best friend may turn out to be your greatest backer on your journey, but it is best to wipe the slate clean and build your team from scratch—if your family and friends want a spot on your team, let them prove to you that they belong there!

Picking Your Team

Time to play detective: It's time to identify the people who are on your Transformation Team, and weed out the people who aren't.

On a separate sheet of paper, list the 10 people closest to you, who may deserve a spot on your Transformation Team. Then make two column headings: On My Team and Not on My Team.

Now, for each individual, answer these questions:

1. Does this person create unnecessary drama or distractions to pull you away from your transformation commitments?
2. Does this person tempt you with triggers from your past?
3. Does this person make comments or make you feel guilty for wanting to change?
4. Does this person refuse to make small changes in their lifestyle to help you reach your goals?

If your answer was no to all of the above questions, place a checkmark in the column On My Team. If your answer was yes to any of the questions, place a checkmark in the column Not on My Team.

People will come in and out of your life for as long as you live. Begin to ask yourself these questions with the people you meet, and determine if they are on your Transformation Team or if they aren't.

Note: Beware the mole! This is the person who pretends to support you on the surface, but as you move closer to your goals, he or she may begin to sabotage you and pull you off course.

If you are having difficulty identifying people to be on your Transformation Team, ask these questions to help guide your search. Your team may be closer than you think!

1. Where might I meet other people who share my goals and attitude toward success?
2. What websites or online communities might connect me with these like-minded people?

And don't forget us and our community of amazing people!

Within your Transformation Team you may find an individual who goes above and beyond motivating and supporting you. They want to see you succeed, and will go the extra mile to help you make it happen. They are there for you to vent, to confess, to open up about your struggles. They also call you out when you are making excuses or trying to rationalize bad behavior. This is your superfriend. Your superfriend tells you what you *need* to hear to better your life, not what you *want* to hear. You may not like what they have to say sometimes (because deep down, you know that they are right). Your superfriend is essential to your success, so it's important to pick this person carefully. Here are some guiding questions to help you:

1. Do I trust this person completely?
2. Do I feel comfortable being totally honest with this person, no matter what I've done?
3. Am I sure that this person will not judge me or get angry with me if I confess a setback?

You and your superfriend must make an agreement between the two of you. Why? Because being a superfriend is not easy. It is a lot easier and much less time consuming to just go along with everything *you* want. Being a superfriend is hard work. Nobody wants to hurt your feelings or for you to be upset with them...but your superfriend cares so much about you, they are willing to tell you the truth even when it might hurt—for *your* success. So take some time to let them know how much you appreciate their sacrifice for you—and that you will stay as open as possible, even when they are calling you out and you are feeling defensive!

If a fight begins, we use a code word to put everything into perspective for both parties. Just say "Superfriend." You'll both know what is happening and remember the agreement you made.

Please share this with your superfriend:

If you are chosen as a superfriend, you must agree to the following:

1. You will call out the individual when you see they are making excuses or justifying destructive behavior.
2. You will listen openly and without judgment when the other individual is confessing.
3. After their confession, the first two words out of your mouth should always be "Thank you."
4. You will be there for support (and maybe even jump into a workout or two) every chance you get.

Creating your Transformation Team is one of the crucial parts of sustaining your motivation, accountability, and perseverance on your transformation journey! Making big changes to how we think and go about our daily routines is very hard. And your Transformation Team is one of the single most important factors in holding you accountable so that you can keep your promises... and create your destiny!

DAY 6

Day 6: Low-Carb Day

Meal 1: Breakfast

    Recipe: Raspberry Almond Oatmeal

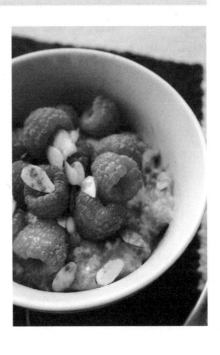

Meal 2: Low-Carb Meal

    Recipe: Chicken Slaw Dip

Meal 3: Low-Carb Meal

    Recipe: Vietnamese Grilled Chicken
Spring Rolls with Sweet Ginger Lime Sauce

Meal 4: Low-Carb Meal

    Recipe: Vanilla Pecan Pudding

Meal 5: Low-Carb Meal

    Recipe: Citrus and Onion Fish Tacos

Day 6: Metabolic Mission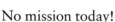

No mission today!

Day 6: Accelerator: 5 minutes (minimum)

Select any activity of your choosing, and keep your heart rate above 120 beats per minute (bpm) the entire time. Prescribed optional interval for maximum results: Mighty Minutes (1:00 low intensity / 1:00 high intensity)

LESSON 6
MAKE IT YOUR OWN!

Never, ever underestimate the importance of having fun.

—Randy Pausch

Setting SMART goals, preparing, and building a trusted Transformation Team all build the foundation for lasting transformation. But we don't want you to forget another extremely important part of your journey: having fun! It is basic common sense: If this new life isn't enjoyable, you aren't going to stick with it.

We've given you the Extreme Transformation structure and plan for success, but now it's time to make it yours—to customize the plan to fit your goals, your needs, your life. How do you do that? By customizing this new lifestyle, rewarding yourself, and trying new ways to make weight loss actually enjoyable.

We mean it: You should be excited about what you are eating and doing. If it isn't fun, then you're doing it wrong. Whether you reach your goal in three short weeks or you are on a yearlong transformation trek, it is important that this process is enjoyable for you. Keep in mind that maintenance—keeping the weight off forever—is very similar to the structure you will follow to lose the weight. So let's make this something you can do forever. Because to keep the weight off, this *is* what you're going to be doing…for life!

The Secret of Substitutions

We mentioned earlier that we designed these 21 days of recipes to give you a plethora of new ideas and concepts for eating and enjoying food as you lose weight. When you try these recipes, we are confident that you will find ones that you absolutely love, and ones that don't suit your palate as much. That's okay! It is all part of the process.

Say you like lean ground beef over ground chicken. No problem, switch them out! Perhaps you prefer Greek yogurt to cottage cheese...plug it in! Maybe you prefer whole-grain pasta over potatoes. So if a recipe calls for potatoes, substitute whole-grain pasta instead! You know what to do—make the switch!

As long as you stay within the Extreme Cycle portions and calorie limits, you can substitute to your heart's content and still achieve the same phenomenal weight loss results.

Reward Yourself!

Motivation is a tricky business. Our brains and bodies are incredibly smart and adapt to new routines easily and quickly. Which is why making changes to our behaviors is so darn hard. One of the ways we can break into our routines to make them more fun and exciting is by giving ourselves rewards. As you've seen, we have designed the Extreme Cycle to include a reward on the seventh day of every week. That means on Days 7, 14, and 21, you will be able to enjoy anything you want, in moderation of course.

The choice of when and what you reward yourself with is up to you! Of course, we wouldn't be Team Powell if we didn't also offer you a list of delicious and nutritious Clean Cheats on Reset days (see page 86 for complete list of Clean Cheats), but in reality you can choose any food you like to be your reward.

There is just one main rule to rewarding yourself: *You cannot reward yourself at or after dinner.* It must always be earlier in the day. In the evening and at night, our inhibitions are down and we are *very* likely to eat more than we should—breaking promises and starting a dangerous backslide. Because of this, any reward should be enjoyed earlier in the day, preferably at or before lunch. Dinner will always remain a sacred low-carb meal, anchoring in your commitment to this journey.

Being able to relax from a routine enables your mind to take a break and restore itself, but here's the best secret: Boosting your calorie intake also boosts your metabolism, so when you drop back into carb cycling on the next day, you will burn even more calories!

For many people, a week is still a pretty darn long time to wait to get your pizza. By the time Wednesday rolls around, it is consuming your thoughts and you can't think of anything else. That's why many people still need what we call Daily Hugs—those little treats that you reward yourself with once or twice a day…just to get you through. We get it. Here's a list of Daily Hugs that you can weave into your daily routine to keep your mind and your taste buds happy until Reset day:

- Diet soda
- Low-calorie specialty coffee
- Calorie-free (or very low-calorie) candy
- Sugar-free gum

Two Heidi Tips

Tip #1 I have found that when I eat such "reward" foods as potato chips or ice cream, I can't stop. It's like my body and brain crave these two foods so intensely, it's near impossible to eat just a little. So my advice is this: Know what your super-trigger foods are and stay away from them. Find a sweet or salty food that you enjoy that doesn't trigger you. Or better yet: Find another pleasurable way to reward yourself—like getting your nails done, getting a massage, or curling up on your couch to watch your favorite show. Rewards are super important, but you still need to be mindful!

Tip #2 To get through the week without feeling any deprivation, I treat myself with one thing every day—I enjoy my own specialty coffee drink—an iced coffee with one pump of mocha and a splash of heavy cream. It has a small calorie impact (less than 100 calories), and it is the Daily Hug that I can look forward to once—or even sometimes twice—every day. It satisfies me enough so that I don't crave anything else…and just look forward to the next morning!

Reward days naturally happen on high-carb days because of their sweet and fatty content. We suggest that Sundays are great for reward days, but it's really up to you. It may make more sense for you to have your reward day (Days 7, 14, and 21 of the Extreme Cycle) on a Wednesday. It's up to you to decide, but you must declare it and commit to it in advance so that you stay clear and focused on your promises to yourself.

Rewards also help you curb your cravings for those trigger foods—sweet, salty, and fatty. But heed this word of caution: Since reward foods can be close to those comfort foods that can trigger overeating (see page 164 for more on identifying your triggers), it's wise to be mindful of your choices. By choosing from our list, you might avoid triggering those old cravings that led to your weight gain to begin with.

Clean Cheat Recipes!

We are not kidding: These Clean Cheat snacks and meals are so delicious (and easy to make), you're going to think we are nuts! They will have your mouth watering and your bellies satisfied. You won't believe they are cleaner versions of those good ol' comfort foods! Just a heads-up, though: The Clean Cheats are cleaner, but please know that they are *still* only acceptable on Reset days, as they are higher in calories than the foods you will be eating on your high- and low-carb days. Check out the recipes in the back section of the book! And remember: Only eat these meals on Days 7, 14, and 21. Bon appétit!

Breakfast

Hootenanny Pancakes
Chocolate Glazed Crepes

Candied Pecan Protein Waffles

Snacks

Spinach Artichoke Dip with Pita Chips
Peanut Butter Chocolate Chip Cookie
   Dough
Muddy Buddies
Sweet Potato Nachos
Homemade Oreos
Banana Berry Ice Cream
Pigs in a Blanket
One-Minute Brownie

Lunch/Dinner

Chunky Monkey Bowl
BLT Burger and Sweet Potato Fries
Barbecue Chicken Pita Pizza
Mac and Cheese with Bacon

If you find yourself craving some typical junk foods, try these amazing substitutions. Often we are simply seeking something that will satisfy our needs for something crunchy, sweet, and/or salty. These should do the trick!

Instead of eating this:	Eat this:
Candy bar or chocolate	Protein bar or shake
Crackers or cookies	Flavored rice cakes
Potato or tortilla chips	Air-popped popcorn
Juice or soda	Calorie-free drink
Pizza	Sliced tomato with low-fat mozzarella, sprinkled with garlic, basil, and sea salt
Ice cream	Sugar-free Popsicle
High-calorie coffee beverage	Iced-coffee with sugar-free syrup
Candy	Sugar-free gum

Heidi Tip

Just like a lot of folks, I get the munchies later in the day, especially after dinner when the kids are in bed and I finally unwind and relax. That's when I often find myself in the "red zone"—that high-alert place where I am craving something sweet or salty. My go-to fix? I put a bag of frozen or fresh broccoli in a bowl, sprinkle a little sea salt or ¼ cup marinara sauce on top, and microwave or steam for a few minutes. This trick not only ups my veggies for the day (always a positive) but also satisfies my cravings! Try it—my peeps have gone crazy for this treat!

Have Fun Accelerating Your Weight Loss!

The key to long-term success is to make exercise enjoyable. If you like doing it, you're going to do it for a long time! If you don't like to do it, you will eventually stop—and go right back to your old habits. Science has found that we are programmed to play—run, jump, push, roll, pull, climb, throw, et cetera—and when we do it in a "gamified" way, the results and benefits are astounding... and fun!

Along these lines, finding the right "Accelerator" for you is a lot like dating. You've got to try them all out to find which ones you love. That's why we encourage everyone to "speed date" every aspect of sport imaginable— brisk walking, rowing, Zumba, running, soccer, basketball, CrossFit, boxing, MMA, whatever! Eventually, you will find something that you truly love to do—even if it's just watching TV while walking on the treadmill. If you enjoy it, then do it to accelerate your weight loss. There is an athlete inside all of us, and we have yet to work with anyone who hasn't found some activity they love.

Cassie rediscovered all the sports she likes. As she told us, "I'm not a gym rat. But for so long when I was overweight, I couldn't play the sports I used to love. Now I play basketball and volleyball. I do some circuit training that I set up in my house. You've just got to get out there and try different things—it's so much more fun than I ever thought."

Part of Merhbod's motivation to stick to his transformation journey was wanting to do everything he used to love—from basketball to skiing. Then he realized that doing those things he used to love was exactly how he'd get back into shape! Granted, moving up and down the court at his heaviest of 434 pounds wasn't easy at first, but he did it anyway. Day after day it got easier and easier, as he lost over 200 pounds and was running circles around his competition!

Bruce discovered CrossFit and now participates in competitions around his region.

David found MMA and trained for 60 to 90 minutes a day, losing over 200 pounds in a year.

Denise picked up tennis and now plays in a competitive doubles league.

Margaret tried Zumba and loves it!

Variety Is the Spice of Life

When we first meet most of our peeps for the show, they seem to fall into two categories—those who love sports and think of themselves as athletes, even if they are now out of shape, and those who say they hate to exercise and would never consider themselves athletes. We are here to tell you that everyone has an athlete inside of them—you just haven't connected with the sport or exercise you love yet. Seriously. We have yet to work with anyone who didn't find something they love to do.

So now is your time! You've got to get out of your comfort zone and let yourself try something new. Take a look at the list below. We challenge you to try something new each of the three weeks of your 21-day cycle. If you don't find something that you really enjoy, keep trying. Your favorite weight-loss Accelerator is out there!

Accelerators

At Home

Dodgeball	Stationary bike	Treadmill
Jump rope	Tag	
Rowing machine	Trampoline	

At the Gym

Arc trainer	Rowing machine	Stationary or recumbent bike
Arm ergometer	Stair stepper	
Elliptical trainer		Treadmill

Outdoors

Bicycling	In-line skating	Stair running
Bleacher running	Jogging/running	Swimming
Canoeing	Kayaking	Walking
Cross-country skiing	Rowing	Water jogging
Hiking	Snow shoveling	
Ice skating	Snowshoeing	

Sports

Basketball	Dodgeball	Hockey
Boxing	Flag football	Jiu Jitsu

Kickball	Racquetball	Tennis
Kickboxing	Soccer	Volleyball
Lacrosse	Squash	Wrestling
Martial arts	Swimming	

Group Classes

Aerobics	CrossFit	Step aerobics
BarSculpt	Dancing	Water aerobics
Cardio kickboxing	Spinning/cycling	

Pick your top five Accelerators from the list above. Choose Accelerators that you already love to do, or have always wanted to try:

Now, here are your marching orders: Do them! Pick one and have some fun with it. If or when it starts to get boring or monotonous, try the next one! Maybe even alternate and switch them up every week. However you do it, have fun!

Become a Metabolic Master

As we described earlier, the way to boost your fat burn to lose even more weight is by including Accelerators into your daily routine. As you move through the 21-day cycles, use this chart of minimum Accelerator times to challenge yourself.

	Week1	Week 2	Week 3
1st Cycle	5 minutes	10 minutes	15 minutes
2nd Cycle	20 minutes	25 minutes	30 minutes
3rd Cycle	35 minutes	40 minutes	45 minutes
4th Cycle	50 minutes	55 minutes	60 minutes

DAY 7

Congrats! You've made it to Day 7: weigh-in and reward day! We are so excited for you! You've already accomplished so much in one short week: You've begun cleaning out your body and your home; you're becoming familiar with your new routine. Now it's time to see the progress.

Weigh In

Weigh in first thing in the morning without eating or drinking. Remove as many articles of clothing as possible to get the cleanest weight.

Your current weight: _____

At this time, feel free to take any other measurements as well and note them here: _____

Day 7: Reset Day

It's Reset Day! Make meals easy by cooking up our Clean Cheat recipes, or simply add 1,000 extra calories of foods you love to a normal high-carb day.

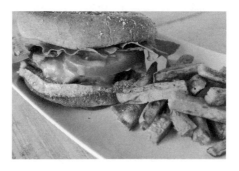

1. Meal 1: Hootenanny Pancakes
2. Meal 2: Spinach Artichoke Dip with Pita Chips
3. Meal 3: Chunky Monkey Bowl
4. Meal 4: BLT Burger and Sweet Potato Fries
5. Meal 5: Peanut Butter Chocolate Chip Cookie Dough

Rest Day

Now relax! Take the day off and rest—no Metabolic Missions and no Accelerators!

LESSON 7
TROUBLESHOOT!

Fall down seven times, get up eight.

—Japanese proverb

As you trek through the days of this journey, you will begin to run into different challenges that can possibly derail you. Sometimes it is the frustration of not losing weight, other times it is uncontrollable cravings. Not to worry—we encounter them on a regular basis and we'll teach you all of the tips and tricks for how to get through them.

Scale Funk

Nothing is worse than working your ass off and seeing no return on the scale. Chillax. If you did it right, you very well may have burned a lot of fat—your body just isn't showing it yet. This reaction is natural and normal. Weight loss may stall for a week or two, but then resume after that.

The body loses fat in slow motion. We recommend you weigh in once a week—the shortest amount of time to see somewhat accurate changes on the scale. We can see a much better trend for weight loss every 2 weeks, but a weekly weigh in promotes accountability and structure. While fat is gained and lost very slowly, water can be gained and lost extremely fast—sometimes we can gain or lose upwards of 10 pounds of water in a day! If you step on the scale every day, these fluctuations can cause an emotional roller coaster. Expect the scale jump up several pounds after every Reset day, then slowly drop over the course of the week. The final 2 low-carb days before the weigh-in, you should see a good drop on the scale, to reveal a clean weight for your weigh-in day.

Here are the four main physiological reasons for seeing a slow loss or even a gain on the scale, as well as some unorthodox ways to get dropping again!

Muscle Swelling

Reason: It occurs to some degree after every Metabolic Mission. The amount of swelling depends upon the intensity of the workout. The higher the intensity, the greater the swelling. This lasts for one to several days, then subsides.

Solutions:

- Reduce the intensity of the Missions for a week; the fluid will release.
- Light massage.
- Epsom salt baths.

Excess Water Retention

Reason A: When sodium intake exceeds the body's normal level, it causes excess water retention and bloat—up to 15 pounds sometimes!

Solution: Reduce your sodium intake and avoid processed, sugary, and salty foods. Drink *lots* of water, and your body will release the excess water over the next three days.

Reason B: Cortisol. This stress hormone is being released in massive amounts from physical stress (overtraining) during long bouts of exercise. The hormone causes fluid retention in the muscles and subcutaneously (under the skin).

Solution: Reduce your training intensity and ensure proper calorie (and carbohydrate) intake. Excess fluid will release over the week and reveal your true loss.

Reason C: Prior dehydration—from not drinking enough water, alcohol consumption, or some other diuretic. The body responds by retaining water.

Solution: Drink at least an extra quart of water daily (aim for at least a gallon daily) and give it three days to stabilize.

Fat Gain or Plateau

Reason: You are consuming too many calories and not burning enough, creating a plateau or even a slow fat and/or muscle *gain*.

Solution: Ensure you are keeping your promises to the Extreme Cycle, Metabolic Missions, and Accelerators. Also, double-check your portions—if you have been simply eyeballing your portions, you may want to pull out the measuring cups for a week to get the portions and calories back on track.

How you can help yourself:

- Are you doing your Accelerators?
- Are you following your commitment to the Extreme Cycle?
- Have you been emotionally eating?

Now is the time to be courageous, open, and honest if you are struggling and eating more than you should. You *may* also be gaining some muscle—especially if you haven't done any form of resistance training in a long time. In the first few weeks of training, it is also common to experience a phenomenon called recomposition: It is when your body gains muscle and loses fat at the same time. This is typically most noticeable in just the first few weeks of training, but can happen subtly over the whole course of your transformation.

Hormonal Fluctuations

Reason A: Women can retain fluid during their monthly cycles. This retention typically lasts no longer than a week.

Reason B: Thyroid, ADH, or Aldosterone fluctuations.

Solution: Bloodwork prescribed by a doctor can determine if this is an issue. It may require medication.

Crush Your Cravings

Every single one of us experiences cravings—for sleep, for water, for sweets, for salty foods, you name it. Cravings are our body's way of telling us *what it thinks* we need. But we are not simple animals roaming the savannas or forests in search of immediate gratification. No. We are thinking beings and we have the power to control our cravings. Obviously, the very first step is by sticking to the Extreme Carb Cycle, exercising regularly, and getting enough sleep.

We also know enough to stay away from our trigger foods and reward ourselves so that we don't make ourselves vulnerable to cravings. But physical cravings can be overwhelming at times, so this is what we recommend:

1. Stay hydrated. Hydration is the number one way to curb cravings. Immediately do our 10-gulp water rule as soon as a craving starts. As soon as

the cup or bottle touches your lips, take 10 gulps before putting it down! It's easy to confuse thirst with hunger, so stay hydrated!

2. Chew sugar-free mint-flavored gum, eat a sugar-free breath mint, or put a dab of toothpaste on your tongue. The mint flavor overwhelms the taste buds, crushing cravings for sweet and salty foods—so you can make it to your next snack or meal.

3. Always include high-fiber foods with breakfast. Fiber-rich foods slow down digestion to keep you fuller for longer, so you will be less likely to overeat later in the day, and more likely to pay attention to your body's signals that it is full.

4. When all else fails, the last resort that is sure to nuke a craving is to use dietary fats, followed by 1 or 2 cups of liquid (water, tea). It takes about 20 minutes after eating the fats for them to close off the valve from the stomach to the intestines. Once you drink the liquid, it fills the stomach, sending an extremely strong "full" signal to the brain, and curbing the strongest of cravings. Warning: The following fats have a 100-calorie impact, so you *must* count it for your daily intake!

A small handful of almonds, then 1 to 2 cups water
1 tablespoon of peanut butter or almond butter, then 1 to 2 cups water
1 stick of string cheese, then 1 to 2 cups water
1 tablespoon of avocado, then 1 to 2 cups water

Or try one of these three delicious 100-calorie liquid treats:

Root beer float: ice-cold diet root beer + 1 tablespoon heavy cream
Coconut water: 1 cup warm water + 1 tablespoon coconut oil
Bulletproof coffee: 1 cup coffee + 1 tablespoon unsalted butter

Again, keep in mind that each of these has a 100-calorie impact, so it must be added to your daily calories. Although we recommend you use the calorie-free methods to curb cravings, if necessary these delicious treats can be used anytime on the Extreme Cycle to curb the heaviest of cravings when they hit. Limit yourself to no more than one per day and sip on it for a while—make it last!

POWELL

LOVE IT!

So where are you now in your journey?

You're building some incredible momentum now after just seven days of Extreme Transformation! You might already be feeling better about yourself, noticing some weight loss and other positive changes in your body. You may feel lighter and cleaner. You may feel more empowered, clearheaded, and centered in yourself. You likely also feel more resolved in your new changes and commitments to yourself.

But as we cautioned you earlier in the book, the diet and exercise plan is the easy part. Just losing weight does not guarantee the deep, life-sustaining transformation we can help create for you.

So for Week Two, we share with you seven more lessons that are crucial to learning to *love* your journey of transformation. These mental and emotional tools will help you dig deep, be vulnerable, and banish the negative self-talk that can derail you. You will, once and for all, conquer your fears, unload the real weight you've been carrying around, and create a new identity that crystallizes your destiny!

DAY 8

Day 8: High-Carb Day

Meal 1: Breakfast
  Recipe: Sweet Potato Fritters

Meal 2: High-Carb Meal
  Recipe: Piña Colada Dream

Meal 3: High-Carb Meal
  Recipe: Chile Relleno, Braised Adobo Chicken, Black Bean and Quinoa Salad

Meal 4: High-Carb Meal
  Recipe: Hulk Shake

Meal 5: Low-Carb Meal
  Recipe: Thai-Style Turkey Cabbage Salad

Day 8: Metabolic Mission: The Grinder (Stepladder)

Set a running clock and, as fast as you can, do 21 reps of each exercise, then do 15 reps of each exercise, then do 9 reps of each exercise. Report your time in your Daily Tracker!

Burpees

Mountain Climbers

Back Lunges

Day 8: Accelerator: 10 minutes (minimum)

Select any activity of your choosing, and keep your heart rate above 120 beats per minute (bpm) the entire time. Prescribed optional interval for maximum results: Dirty Two-Thirties (2:30 low intensity / 2:30 high intensity)

LESSON 8
BELIEVE IN YOURSELF

Whether you think you can or whether you think you can't, you're right.

—Henry Ford

Yes, the promises you make to yourself are concrete, convincing accomplishments. But often people feel terrified, doubtful, and just plain confused as they begin to make even the smallest of changes. In fact, beginning and sticking to this journey requires a certain "leap of faith," which often feels like moving into unknown territory. This is where you need a little faith. Faith in this process, and faith in all the people who have succeeded before you. Because if they can do it, you can do it.

But sometimes believing in yourself isn't easy, and that's where we come in.

We know you are capable of this journey. We know that it's not easy. But it is possible. As Bruce shared with us, "Chris and Heidi, I needed you. At first I didn't know if I could do it, but you helped me believe in myself again. Your support and love helped me realize that I can do this. Once I started to believe in myself, I'd say, *I'm not going to let the fat beat me today.* And you know what, it didn't. I just needed to believe!"

Our work with thousands of overweight people who have lost thousands of pounds has shown us one truth over and over again: One of the most powerful ingredients to changing your life is simply believing that you can. Seems overly simplistic, but actually getting you to *believe* in your abilities—to know in your heart of hearts that you can do this—can be a difficult task.

Belief is the magic ingredient that drives your choices and behaviors. When you believe, the light switch for transformation gets slammed into the "on" position and you excitedly put forth the effort to achieving your goals and dreams. The moment you question yourself or stop believing that you can, the switch slams off. And just as quickly, your behaviors can revert back to their old habits and patterns.

But what if you've tried and failed what seems like hundreds of times in the past?

What if you don't think that you can attain your goal?

There are a couple of ways to develop belief when you don't believe in yourself...yet.

This new commitment to transformation requires courage in the face of past experience and failures. How many diets have you tried? How many have worked for you? How many times have you gone through a dieting ordeal only to end up gaining the weight back and feeling like a failure, ashamed of your inability to succeed or stick with it?

Let us help put any doubts you have to rest. Seeing is believing. One of the most powerful sources of inspiration is seeing another person we can relate to accomplish extraordinary goals. That's why every year we select 15 to 20 new and unique individuals to embark upon the journey of transformation. As we often tell our peeps, we love working with them because they have such a long and challenging journey ahead—the literal sizes of their journeys to weight loss are daunting for almost anyone to imagine. However, time and time again they do it. They finish their yearlong journey and they just keep going. We document their journey and share it across the world so that everyone can see what we as humans are capable of. We love working with our people, because they leave no doubt on the table that anyone and everyone can change for the better.

Why are we sharing this? Because if they can do it, so can you. They not only learned to trust the process and go all in, but they came to believe in themselves.

You can trust the thousands of people who have reached their successful weight loss goals using Extreme Transformation—its eating, exercise plan, and lessons. So now it is your time. Just take a look at the before-and-after photos below.

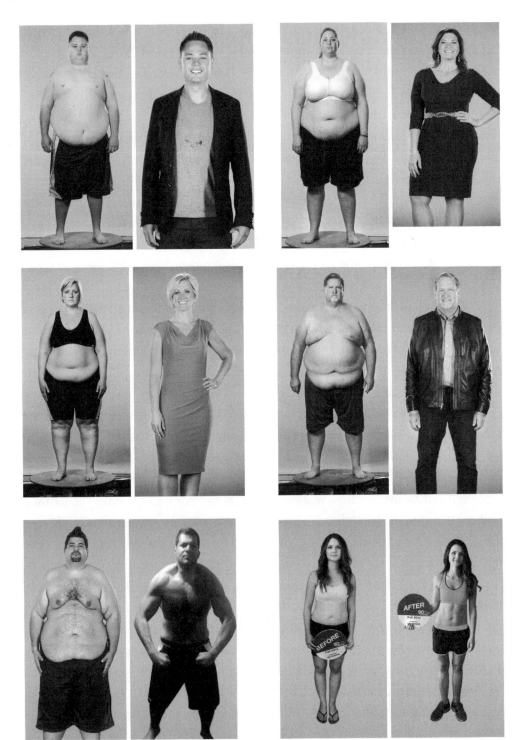

These amazing transformations are a testament to what you are also capable of.

Call to Action: Learning How to Believe in Yourself

Begin by writing down three accomplishments that you are proud of having achieved in your life:

1.

2.

3.

Next, name three people whose lives you have helped:

1.

2.

3.

Consider these accomplishments. Reflect on them. Take pride in them. You need to remind yourself of what you have achieved.

It's possible to tap into the extraordinary—just like Bruce, Cassie, Jeff, Georgeanna, Mehrbod, and the thousands of others who have chosen to believe in themselves. We believe that though we are all ordinary humans, we all have the ability to be extraordinary. But you have to believe it's possible. Without that belief as your source, you simply will not put forward the energy and perseverance to get there.

Remember—it's okay if you don't believe in yourself yet. Turn to your Transformation Team, turn to us, turn to your online support group! Borrow their belief in you until you feel it for yourself!

Know this truth…we believe in you, we're excited for you, and we know you are going to do extraordinary things.

DAY 9

Day 9: High-Carb Day

Meal 1: Breakfast
> Recipe: Banana Yogurt Parfait and
Pumpkin Seed Granola

Meal 2: High-Carb Meal
> Recipe: Egg Salad on Toast

Meal 3: High-Carb Meal
> Recipe: Green Chili Turkey and Cilantro Rice Bowl

Meal 4: High-Carb Meal
> Recipe: Peanut Butter Shake

Meal 5: Low-Carb Meal
> Recipe: Salmon with Pesto "Zoodles"

Day 9: Metabolic Mission: Runnin' Wild (RFT)

Set a running clock and do 7 rounds of the following circuit as fast as you can. Record your time in your Daily Tracker!

10 Burpees
15 Sit-Ups
25 High Knees

Day 9: Accelerator: 10 minutes (minimum)

Select any activity of your choosing, and keep your heart rate above 120 beats per minute (bpm) the entire time. Prescribed optional interval for maximum results: Thrilling Thirties (:30 low intensity / :30 high intensity)

LESSON 9
BE OPEN, HONEST, AND VULNERABLE

Vulnerability is the greatest marker of courage.

—Brené Brown

On Day 1 of our boot camp, we face our new group of participants and shock them to their very core. They are expecting hugs, high-fives, and for us to immediately start talking about all the weight they are going to lose. They are hoping, praying, and expecting that we give them the golden ticket of diet and exercise advice. They believe these are the true tools to changing their lives! But as you probably understand by now, true transformation actually has very little to do with diet and exercise, and everything to do with the deep, meaningful steps that truly alter your being.

So on that first day, we open the kimono. We explain that transformation has little to do with how you eat and move, and much more to do with how open, honest, and vulnerable you are willing to be. When we are vulnerable, we can grow. We can change.

Are you ready to let go and be truly vulnerable? Because that's what it's going to take. There's some tough love ahead...

Our Need for Connection

It is human nature to seek acceptance from others—in fact, belonging is an inherent drive or need that all humans have. We all must feel loved and accepted in order to feel whole and complete. We are social animals and therefore we are "interdependent" and need help and cooperation from others for our very survival. In response to this drive, many of us—beginning when we are small children—begin to develop what we think is a "better" version of ourselves— a version that we feel is more lovable and acceptable than who we *really* are inside. This version of you strives to look its very best in front of others. This is the version that lied when you were younger so that people wouldn't think less of you. It is the version that tells everyone how well you are doing, when deep down inside you know you are struggling. It is the version that hides the donuts from the break room in its desk drawer for later—because it doesn't want to look weak in front of its co-workers. It is the version that *swears* it is doing everything right, when in reality it knows that it is breaking its promises left and right. It cannot handle embarrassment or the thought of being rejected. As we get older, that barrier becomes thicker and harder.

But this protective barrier comes at a huge cost. It is totally inauthentic, and deep down...you know it. The life you are living is a complete fraud. And even worse, because it is inauthentic, you feel like nobody could possibly love the "real you"—who you *really* are—and nobody knows how you *really* feel. You feel like you must carry on this facade, this front, forever. If you don't, you fear you will be unlovable.

Well, you're wrong. In fact, letting down this barrier is what opens your heart and mind for lifelong change—and will make you more lovable than ever!

Georgeanna, a self-described perfectionist, was unable to see herself as anything but the perfect person she thought she had to be in order to be loved. But the real Georgeanna had become over 100 pounds overweight, living two separate existences—the one in her head where she still thought she had to be a perfect mother, wife, daughter, and the one who walked around during the day, a ghost of her real self. Where was the real Georgeanna? Buried. Muted.

Georgeanna's biggest step was seeing herself naked and having the courage to say, "This is who I am right now."

Georgeanna remembers the exact moment I had her disrobe and step on the scale in front of her family and friends. She never felt more vulnerable in her entire life. She had never, ever shared how much she weighed with her husband, Scott, or anyone else in her life—let alone her whole community. She put all of her energy into doing good work for others (her "perfect" self), as if to erase the reality that she had an enormous weight problem and food addiction.

So with all the courage she could muster, Georgeanna stepped on the scale. What happened next was the exact opposite of what she thought would happen. Instead of people snickering and laughing, they began to applaud. They shouted words of encouragement and love. This first step unleashed a torrent of tears...followed by a torrent of successes. Her ability to let herself be so vulnerable paved the way for her to confront her fears, give herself permission, and ultimately declare what she wanted: weight loss, health, and a chance to change the way she was living that was making her so unhappy with herself. She realized that she could be open and honest with everyone about her mistakes and slip-ups along the way, not having to report that she was doing everything perfectly all the time—and everyone loved her *more* because of it. As she told us, "I would lie down at night and feel proud of myself and the choices I made throughout the day—instead of feeling ashamed, afraid, and filled with dread and self-loathing."

In that moment of vivid vulnerability, Georgeanna's authentic self was revealed and she was able to summon the courage to move forward into her real journey. If she hadn't allowed herself to become that open and vulnerable, she would not have succeeded.

To put our mind into a place where we are open to change, we must be truly "authentic." We must be wholly open and honest with ourselves, and with others.

To be authentic, we need to understand our ego. Our ego is the protective barrier we were speaking of earlier. It was built to protect us, but most often hinders our ability for growth and change. Embracing your ego and the role that it plays enables you to put it aside and get on with your *real* life.

So what does it take to be vulnerable? Sometimes it is a physical step like disrobing and looking in a mirror or stepping on a scale. Sometimes it's more the emotional step of being truly honest about your imperfections, and sharing openly with others about your fears, your mistakes, your dreams and aspirations. This is all part of being human that most of us hide, but being vulnerable is the only way to truly change and grow. Let yourself be truly honest about who you are. This creates the clearing for an open mind and growth. And you very well may be surprised…your vulnerability gives others around you permission to also open up for healing and growth!

Call to Action: Step on the Scale

It doesn't matter if you're 160 pounds or 560 pounds; if you have avoided stepping on the scale earlier, it's time. It's time to be open, honest, and vulnerable with yourself. Strip down and step on the scale. Then face yourself in the mirror.

1. Write down what it feels like to see the number on the scale (for maybe the first time), what it feels like to be naked in front of the mirror, and what it feels like to face yourself in the mirror.

2. Get the feelings out. They've only been holding you back. What do you feel when you see yourself and your weight?

3. Now say good-bye to that number on the scale, and say good-bye to the old you. You have a bright, healthy, and fit future ahead, and now you are well on your way to getting there!

Heidi Tip

As a woman, stepping on the scale is naturally tough for me, especially having battled an eating disorder for most of my teenage years and early adulthood! But the more I do it, and the more I push myself to get comfortable with being uncomfortable, the easier it gets… and the more I love and accept myself for who I am. So don't fear the scale. Let it simply be a tool to help you stay honest and accountable.

DAY 10

Day 10: High-Carb Day

Meal 1: Breakfast
    Recipe: Huevos Rancheros

Meal 2: High-Carb Meal
    Recipe: PB & J Rice Cakes and Shake

Meal 3: High-Carb Meal
    Recipe: Grilled Ginger Lime Tuna and Steamed Vegetable Medley

Meal 4: High-Carb Meal
    Recipe: Triple Berry Treat

Meal 5: Low-Carb Meal
    Recipe: Pepper Jack Chicken

Day 10: Metabolic Mission: Mt. Everest (Chipper)

Set a running clock and complete one round of this circuit as fast as you can. Record your time in your Daily Tracker!

20 Burpees
30 Push-Ups
40 Flutterkicks
50 Air Squats
60 Mountain Climbers
70 High Knees

Day 10: Accelerator: 10 minutes (minimum)

Select any activity of your choosing, and keep your heart rate above 120 beats per minute (bpm) the entire time. Prescribed optional interval for maximum results: Tenacious Twos (2:00 low intensity / 2:00 high intensity)

LESSON 10
UNLOAD THE REAL WEIGHT

The weak can never forgive. Forgiveness is an attribute of the strong.
Mahatma Gandhi

Hurt. Vengeance. Sadness. Regret. Rage. We all carry emotional weight on our shoulders...some more than others. Different events in our lives when we were betrayed, hurt, abandoned—or hurt and abandoned others—can haunt us and influence the way we feel about ourselves. These emotions deeply affect our decision making every day. All of these feelings can be categorized into the two major destructive emotions: anger and shame.

Frequently we hear that people who go through massive rehabilitation, like recovery from alcohol, drug, or other addictions, often have to confront a lot of emotional pain or trauma from their past in order to finally find peace. This kind of emotional healing is critical for recovery from addiction if one wants to truly and powerfully change one's life.

However, dealing with this emotional weight is not exclusive to individuals struggling with heavy addictions. We *all* have emotional weight that we carry that is holding us back! Many times we have gone so long carrying the weight that we've almost forgotten that it is there…almost. It's like living life with the flu and forgetting what it is like to feel energetic and healthy. If we want to release this parking brake that is holding us back, we need to unload the real weight!

When Bruce first embarked on his journey of transformation he was motivated by his desire to be a more powerful, active football coach for his young players. He knew that his weight was killing him. But what he did not realize until he was knee-deep into the process is that the shame, emotions, and feelings from his past were preventing him from moving on to the future he dreamed of. He realized that in order to move on, he needed to heal from his own pain suffered at the hands of his father. During our time with Bruce, he admitted that his father had sexually and emotionally abused him for years, since he'd been a little boy. His father was now in prison on multiple counts of sexually molesting other children. But Bruce had never spoken aloud that he, too, was one of his father's victims. The shame of his silence was the real source of what was killing Bruce.

Fortunately, Bruce had an opportunity to unload the weight of his shame and anger when his father came up for parole. Afraid and shaken, Bruce summoned every bit of his courage and confronted his father in a courtroom, telling the parole hearing judge that he was also a victim and that for the safety of him and other children, his father should stay behind bars. Even in this difficult moment, Bruce told his father that he forgave him, and was ready to move on with his life—free from the control of his memories.

From that moment on, Bruce has been unstoppable. He lost weight faster than ever. He got fitter than ever. He worked himself out of debt and started dating. He unloaded the real weight—released the parking brake that had been stuck on for years—and is now living a limitless life, at half of his original body weight. Oh, and now we work side by side with him as one of our incredible transformation coaches!

Take a look at what some of our courageous people unloaded to transform:

- Cassandra chose to forgive herself for giving up her son for adoption and explained to him her wishes for his better life.
- Melissa chose to forgive her late husband for taking his life and abandoning her and her sons.
- Jeff chose to forgive himself for being an absent father and apologized to his family.
- Kenny chose to forgive himself for quitting the marines.
- David chose to forgive himself for not being there for his younger brother and sister when they needed him most.

These were all events and emotions that each of these individuals kept secret or buried for years. Whether it was hurt they endured, or the hurt they caused someone else, unable to deal with the emotions, they numbed themselves with food. It *cost* them, just like it may be costing you right now.

Sound familiar?

What happened? It is a powerful question we ask everyone going through transformation, because once we can identify it, we can help set you free. Here are some experiences that can create a legacy of destructive emotions that will hold you back:

- Death
- Affair
- Molestation
- Abandonment
- Bullying
- Disappointments or failures
- Sexuality
- Segregation
- Sexual assault
- Domestic violence
- Divorce
- Adoption

If you have experienced any of these, you are certainly not alone. In fact, we don't know of anyone who *hasn't* been through at least one of the traumatic events listed above. Whatever side you have been on, these major life events can cause devastating emotions of shame and anger that can, and will, prevent you from achieving your best life and body.

Keep in mind that clearing the past and unloading the weight doesn't mean that you have to forget. It doesn't mean that you are a doormat to get walked on and abused. Clearing the past is for *you* to heal and move on in *your* journey through life. That weight is not yours to carry anymore.

Call to Action: Unloading the Weight

So how can we free ourselves from these destructive emotions and live a limitless life? There is a way . . . let us show you how.

1. Make amends with the past: Create a list of people you have wronged in the past, or people who have wronged *you*. Write down what happened.

2. By yourself in front of a mirror, practice forgiving those people or apologizing to them (and forgiving yourself). Notice we say to *practice* forgiveness. This is because true and authentic forgiveness can take time. It doesn't always happen immediately. Forgiveness can happen over days, weeks, months, and even years. You will likely feel the pain and hurt for a while still, but if you keep practicing, it *will* get better—we promise. Practicing forgiveness is simple: It is wishing other people (or yourself) *peace*. That's it. You don't have to shower them with love and affection, you don't have to be their friend or spend time with them. Just genuinely wish them peace from what happened. It is very likely that they are dealing with their own shame or anger.

3. When you are ready, rally your superfriend or team. Let them know what happened and how you feel about it. Now is a good time to lean on them for emotional support.

4. As long as it will not do any harm to yourself or others (and only if you are truly ready), write a letter, place a phone call, text, email, what have you, to the people on your list, and practice forgiving them, or apologizing to them (and forgiving yourself). If you're not ready yet, feel free to burn the letter, or write and then delete the email.

NOTE: Remember, forgiveness is for *you,* but you will not be set free until your intentions are authentic and you genuinely *feel* it. This is not an easy process, and is one of the most difficult aspects of transformation, but this final step of unloading the weight is extremely powerful and could be the most pivotal moment in changing your life and your body!

Stay attuned to yourself, your feelings, and your triggers. Whenever you begin to experience those shameful or angry feelings, find your superfriend or someone you can confide in openly. Fear of losing connection with others fuels these emotions, so it takes the interaction with another human—to see that you are still lovable—to heal the shame.

Reflection

Again, you may or may not be ready to confront experiences in your past that are painful and causing you shame or anger. We don't want to rush you, and we are certainly not judging you. Simply be aware of what's happened to you, what you have done to someone else, or what you might have witnessed. However, regardless of what has happened, there tends to be a moment (or a few moments) that greatly changed the way you see yourself and the world. Know that if there was no closure to this event (or events), then they will continue to weigh on your mind and hold you back from reaching your greatest potential.

You might also try to identify the source of that feeling you have that "something's wrong with me," or why you feel "different" or "all alone." These inner experiences of detachment, discomfort, and a general sense of not being good enough are common among all of us. You are not alone. When you are ready, come back to this chapter and work through it. You won't regret it.

You will know when the time is right to confront traumatic issues of the past. Being ready is a process and it's one you cannot do alone. So reach out to your team, a therapist, or a self-help group. If you're not ready right now, that's okay. Remember, this is your journey. When you are ready to move forward with no restraints, then you know what to do.

DAY 11

Day 11: High-Carb Day

Meal 1: Breakfast

    Recipe: Hot Quinoa Cereal with Banana

  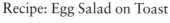

Meal 2: High-Carb Meal

    Recipe: Egg Salad on Toast

Meal 3: High-Carb Meal

    Recipe: Grilled Greek Chicken Kebabs

Meal 4: High-Carb Meal

    Recipe: Lemon Poppy Seed Protein Bites

Meal 5: Low-Carb Meal

    Recipe: Almond-Crusted Tilapia with Asparagus and Cauliflower Mash

Day 11: Metabolic Mission: Hustle Time (AMRAP)

Set a running clock and do as many rounds of the following circuit as possible in 6 minutes.

5 Burpees
7 Mountain Climbers
9 Squats

Day 11: Accelerator: 10 minutes (minimum)

Select any activity of your choosing, and keep your heart rate above 120 beats per minute (bpm) the entire time. Prescribed optional interval for maximum results: Nasty Nineties (1:30 low intensity / 1:30 high intensity)

LESSON 11
BANISH THE NEGATIVE SELF-TALK

If we talked to our friends in the same way that we talk to ourselves, we wouldn't have any friends.

—Anonymous

You know that annoying voice in our heads that relentlessly reminds us that we could have done better or should work harder? The voice that berates us, tells us that we are not smart enough or that we are too fat? We have all, at one time or another, heard this voice of negativity of all that we aren't, all that is wrong with us, and all that is just not good enough.

Does any of this sound familiar?

"I knew I couldn't do it—I am such a loser."
"I am nothing compared with those people."
"I'm such an idiot; I can't believe I'm so stupid."
"I'm no good."
"I am bad."
"I am a failure."
"I am a terrible parent."
"I am worthless."
"Everyone else is better than me."
"I could never do that."

"I'm a monster."
"I'll never be any good at it."
"It's always my fault."
"Nobody likes me."
"I'm not popular."
"I can't cope."

We're going to shoot straight here: This kind of negative thinking brings absolutely nothing good to your life. In fact, it *costs* you joy, confidence, happiness, and ultimately the life (including the body) you want.

In this step, you are going to learn how to control that negative self-talk, to make it work for you—not against you. You are going to destroy that broken record, bury the conversation, and learn how to say affirming and empowering things to yourself. Why is this so important? Because the way we think, literally the content of our thoughts, affects how we feel and act. Behavioral researchers have shown that of the 50,000 or so thoughts we have each and every day, most are automatic, which means they pass through our minds without our realizing it. And if these thoughts are negative or self-critical, then they actually harm our confidence, our beliefs, our self-esteem, and our ability to make beneficial choices through the day.

We are asking you to make big changes to your behaviors. But before you can do that, it's critical that you first stop the barrage of negative, self-denigrating thoughts that are making you think that you can't change, that you can't succeed, and that you can't stick with it.

As humans, what we repeatedly and automatically say to ourselves becomes the foundation for our beliefs. Then it's a matter of time before these negative self-beliefs become a self-fulfilling prophecy. As the saying goes,

"Your thoughts become words, your words become actions, your actions become character, your character becomes your destiny."

In other words, when you find yourself saying negative things about yourself—in your head or out loud—you will begin to act in ways that seem to make such beliefs true.

Letting Go of the Negative

Now is the time to deal with your mind. We are who we tell ourselves we are. Unfortunately, most of the time we are only telling ourselves how unlovable, unacceptable, inadequate, and imperfect we are. We have the hardest time seeing the good within ourselves, and tend to feel guilt when we do! Because so much of our thoughts and brain power is directed toward belittling ourselves, we do eventually become what we feel is an unlovable, unacceptable, inadequate, imperfect person. The good news is that, if we can talk ourselves into being inadequate, we can also talk ourselves into being wonderful, beautiful, powerful, and strong! We have the power to redirect our thoughts and use them to reinforce our goals. How? By replacing negative, self-sabotaging ways of thinking with positive, affirming, and dignity-inspired thoughts.

Identifying your negative thinking is the first step toward creating a positive mindset. The go-to experts in this field are cognitive behaviorists, and they have identified common types of negative thinking. There is overlap among them, but giving each type a name makes it easier to remember them. (If you do any more reading in cognitive therapy, you may come across the term *distorted thinking.* Some authors use that term instead of *negative thinking,* which we think sounds harsh. But we must say, distorted thinking feels so much more accurate because all of the negative things you are saying about yourself, simply aren't true!)

The Big Five Types of Distorted Thinking

Just to prove to you that you are not alone, hundreds of books and thousands of articles have been written on negative thinking and how to turn it around. Why? Because as humans, we *all* do it! In fact, there are textbook categories for all of the thoughts that flow through your head on a daily basis. So to sum it up: Welcome to the club. Now, just like training a muscle, we can train our minds to turn that negative talk into something that doesn't hurt us, but actually helps us! (Source: www.cognitivetherapyguide.org.)

- **All-or-Nothing Thinking/Polarizing**—"I have to do things perfectly, because anything less than perfect is a failure." All-or-nothing thinking is the most common type of negative thinking, and leads to anxiety because you think that any mistake is a failure, which may expose you to criticism or judgment. Therefore you don't give yourself permission to even attempt many things if you don't feel you can do them perfectly. Or if you do attempt, you may tend to lie and hide any mistakes. You are terrified to be vulnerable and honest with yourself. You let your ego stand in the way of you and your authentic self.

- **Disqualifying the Positives/Filtering**—"Life feels like one disappointment after another."
- **Negative Self-Labeling**—"I feel like a failure. I'm flawed. If people knew the real me, they wouldn't like me."
- **Catastrophizing**—"If something is going to happen, it'll probably be the worst-case scenario."
- **Personalizing**—"It's always my fault." When something bad occurs, you automatically blame yourself. For example, you hear that an evening out with friends is canceled, and you assume that the change in plans is because no one wanted to be around you.

Other Common Types of Distorted Thinking

- **Mind Reading**—"I can tell people don't like me because of the way they act around me."
- **Should Statements**—"People should be fair. If I'm nice to them, they should be nice back."
- **Excessive Need for Approval**—"I can only be happy if people like me. If someone is upset, it's probably my fault."
- **Disqualifying the Present**—"I'll relax later. But first I have to rush to finish this."
- **Dwelling on Pain**—"If I dwell on why I'm unhappy and think about what went wrong, maybe I'll feel better." Alternatively, "If I worry enough about my problem, maybe I will feel better."
- **Pessimism**—"Life is a struggle. I don't think we are meant to be happy. I don't trust people who are happy. If something good happens in my life, I usually have to pay for it with something bad."

Call to Action

Go through the different kinds of distorted self-talk, and determine which one you use. Write it/them here: _____

Flip the Switch: Turning the Negative into Positive

So after years of berating ourselves and beating ourselves up, how can we take this continuous conversation and change it? While we covered the power of forgiveness in the last lesson, reversing negative self-talk requires another powerful emotion: appreciation. We have seen most of our people silence these negative voices in their heads and replace them with positive, affirming, empowering voices—using appreciation. Remember, as bad as it seems life can get, there is always someone worse off. There are people in this world that are struggling through war, famine, drought, disease, severe poverty, and the list goes on. A large portion of the world's population is just trying to make it through today alive.

When you think about it, you've got a lot going for you. If you're reading this book, you're literate. And you could actually afford to buy it! You are making strides toward a better you. Let's tap into some "appreciation" and build this list even further:

- **Identify Areas to Change**—First, identify areas of your life that you typically think negatively about, whether it's work, your daily commute, or a relationship. Start small by focusing on just one of those areas to approach in a more positive way. When you say something negative, challenge yourself to think of at least one positive to go with it. Practice appreciation for what you *do* have going for you.
- **Check Yourself**—Periodically during the day, stop and evaluate what you're thinking. If you find that your thoughts are mainly negative, try to find a way to put a positive spin on them. Once again, practice appreciation for yourself and what is working in your life.
- **Be Open to Humor**—Give yourself permission to smile or laugh,

especially during difficult times. Seek humor in everyday happenings. When you can laugh at life, you feel less stressed.

- **Surround Yourself with Positive People**—Rely on your team. You created this positive, empowering network of people—surround yourself with them!
- **Practice Positive Self-Talk**—Start by following one simple rule: Don't say anything to yourself that you wouldn't say to anyone else. Be gentle and encouraging with yourself. If a negative thought enters your mind, evaluate it rationally and respond with affirmations of what is good about you.

One of the most touching and impactful experiences we've ever had with banishing negative self-talk was with Jayce. When we first met Jayce, he was a broken man. He had always been overweight, unathletic, and considered himself a worthless failure. He had recently been through an awful divorce with a verbally abusive ex-wife who berated him daily, making him feel even more worthless. When we started the process of transformation with him, he was down, depressed, and had no confidence that he could actually do it. He couldn't get out of his head the idea that he was a worthless failure—that he didn't deserve this opportunity and that he was going to fail and disappoint everyone.

The bright spot in Jayce's life was his 10-year-old son, whom he loved with all his heart. We sent Jayce home after just a few weeks of boot camp to straighten out some issues back home, and think about if he wanted to return. He chose to come back reluctantly, feeling that he had to. Jayce's mother and his son came to the airport to see him off. In the airport as he was walking toward his plane back to boot camp, his son called out his name and said, "Hey, Dad!"

When Jayce turned around, his son said to him, "You deserve this."

That moment changed everything. Jayce landed at boot camp a totally different man. His son completely flipped Jayce's negative thinking—into a positive conversation that he had with himself every single day. Jayce is now a new man. Twelve months later and 200 pounds lost is proof!!

Here are some examples (source: Mayo Clinic) of negative self-talk and how you can apply a positive twist to them:

Negative Self-Talk	Positive Thinking
I've never done it before.	I love learning new things.
It's too complicated.	I'm creative. I'll tackle it from a different angle.
I don't have the resources.	I'm resourceful. I can find a way to make it happen.
I'm too lazy to get this done.	I'm committed. I wasn't able to fit it into my schedule, but I can reexamine some priorities.
There's no way it will work.	I can make it work. I'll just stay flexible in my approach.
It's too radical a change.	Let's have some fun. Let's take a chance.
No one bothers to communicate with me.	I'll see if I can open the channels of communication.
I'm not going to get any better at this.	I persevere. I'll keep trying until I get it done. Or at least I'll get a helluva lot stronger in the process!

Call to Action: Make Your Own List!

Make two columns. In one, write down all the negative phrases you've used in the past; in the next, write down all the same thoughts but using positive terminology. Follow the example above. Become conscious and aware of your negative feelings and thoughts about yourself and then read aloud the positive affirmations. If you do this regularly, every day for a few weeks, your thinking will begin to shift from negative to positive. You will begin to hear the true inner voice that speaks of your accomplishments, achievements, and love.

Negative	Positive

DAY 12

Day 12: Low-Carb Day

Meal 1: Breakfast
   Recipe: Apple Cinnamon Muesli

Meal 2: Low-Carb Meal
   Recipe: Deviled Eggs

Meal 3: Low-Carb Meal
   Recipe: Chicken Basil Spaghetti

Meal 4: Low-Carb Meal
   Recipe: Chocolate Chip Almond Coconut Bites and Shake

Meal 5: Low-Carb Meal
   Recipe: Cajun Salmon with Cabbage Salad and Steamed Broccoli

Day 12: Metabolic Mission: Breakthrough (Tabata)

For each exercise, do as many reps as you can in 20 seconds. Rest for 10 seconds, then do as many reps as you can in 20 seconds again. Repeat for 8 total rounds (for a total of 4 minutes) per exercise. The lowest number of reps you get in any round is your score. You'll get one score per exercise. Add up all three scores, and record it in your Daily Tracker!

Burpees
Back Lunges
Hollow Rocks

Day 12: Accelerator: 10 minutes (minimum)

Select any activity of your choosing, and keep your heart rate above 120 beats per minute (bpm) the entire time. Prescribed optional interval for maximum results: Mighty Minutes (1:00 low intensity / 1:00 high intensity)

LESSON 12
CREATE YOUR NEW IDENTITY

First say to yourself what you would be; and then do what you have to do.

—Epictetus

Who are you?

It's not a trick question, but the way you answer it will most likely have a lasting impact on your future.

Our identity says a lot about us. Our identity is defined as "the character, qualities, beliefs, etcetera, that make a particular person or group different from another." Character, qualities, beliefs. These are the components of our transformation mind-set! These are what control your choices now and the choices you make in the future. Which is why the way you think about yourself *right now* is critical to your long-term success.

As you move through these steps of transformation, your body will begin to change significantly. As it does so, however, the way you view yourself must change, too—if this transformation is going to last.

The purpose of this lesson is to help you identify the new you. The *real* you. Sometimes this new identity is tied to an aspiration, and sometimes it is linked to a younger self. Either way, it is a brand-new way of defining who you are from the inside out—from the way you act toward others, to the choices you make, to the clothes you wear. In fact, many of our peeps literally change their careers! This lesson is all about realizing who you can *be*, then becoming that person now!

Think about it.

Here's some quick and hard-hitting common sense to put things into perspective for you: If you see yourself as a loser, a disappointment, or a failure, then when faced with everyday decisions in life, you will make the choices of a loser, a disappointment, or failure. We're going out on a limb here, but chances are that those choices will not benefit your health, fitness, and long-term weight loss goals. In short, if you believe this *identity* is you, you will unintentionally choose actions that support that belief.

The same applies for the reciprocal: When you see yourself *now* as a winner, an inspiration, an achiever, a hard worker, and an athlete, that is *exactly* who you'll become.

Two people sit down at a restaurant to order a meal. One is a fat slob, and the other is a world-class athlete. What do they order?

Your meal choices for each would likely differ, wouldn't they? You may think that the fat slob would order something like a cheeseburger and fries, or maybe pizza, right? And the world-class athlete would order chicken and rice, or maybe fish and a baked potato, right?

Here's the trick to the scenario—if that's what you think they'll eat, then that's what they'll eat. So which one are you?

However you see yourself, your actions will support and you will further anchor yourself into that identity! See yourself as a fat slob, and you will become more of a fat slob. See yourself as a world-class athlete and you will become more and more of a world-class athlete!

In this process, we are *being* with the end in mind. We declare who it is that we want to be, then we become that person *now!* Every successive day we live into that new inevitable future—of being a winner, an inspiration, an achiever, a hard worker, and an athlete!

When we immediately become who it is we want to be, negative talk disappears, and positive thinking begins…because the new you, the *real* you, would *never* talk to yourself that way! When faced with decisions, you make choices that positively affect your long-term future, because that is who you are and what you do!

Bruce explains his new identity this way: "My whole life is different now. It took me a while before I understood that I'm not a loser who failed at life. I'm a role model. I'm a coach. I'm an inspiration, and I'm the hardest worker in the room. That's who I chose to be at the beginning of my journey, and that's exactly who I became. I want to help others now. I want to pay it forward."

For Melissa, her new identity emerged more subtly. As she told us, "I wasn't used to being successful in my life." Melissa's new identity was more an internal shift as she became used to feeling differently in her body—more confident and more comfortable. For years, Jami believed she was a monster. When she realized that she is a talented, beautiful inspiration…everything changed.

How Some of Our Peeps Created New Identities

- Bruce left "fat boy" behind and became a CrossFit athlete.
- Melissa abandoned her identity as a fat and lonely widow, and became an inspirational mom to her community.
- Julianna said good-bye to the troubled, tentative teenager and became a fierce role model for her peers.

- Kenny left his discharge from the military behind and once again became a proud U.S. Marine.
- Mike left the sick old man in his past and became the superhero to his kids that he'd always dreamed of being.

What about you?

Call to Action: Who Do You Want to Be?

Go through this quick exercise here or in your journal:

1. Identify your goal.
2. What are the emotional, physical, and lifestyle characteristics of a person who has achieved this goal?
3. What do you need to change about yourself or your life to become this person?
4. Who do you know who has achieved this goal or shares your goal?

Now, it's time to declare your new identity. Describe your new detailed character traits.

_____

_____

_____

_____

_____

_____

Now go back and read what you wrote a few times. All you have to do now, is live *into* this new you.

This "new you" may be a difficult reality to accept, but just try it out. Creating your new identity can be an amazing and powerful experience. For some it clicks right away and they never look back. Others need to practice being that person for a while until the new sense of self sinks in. Just like training muscles, many people need to train their minds to accept positive, empowering images of the self.

Begin right now and try believing it for the next 30 seconds...

Now, while you are this person, write it down:

I am_____

_____.

Great job. Now try it again for 30 more seconds.

As you face life's daily decisions of what to eat, whether or not to exercise, and what to do in certain circumstances, try out your new identity for just a few seconds at a time and see how it feels. Over time, the seconds will become minutes, which will become hours, and then days. You will realize that this new person is exactly who you will become and who you are.

DAY 13

Day 13: Low-Carb Day

Meal 1: Breakfast
    Recipe: "Loaded" Breakfast Potato

Meal 2: Low-Carb Meal
    Recipe: Edamame and Pistachio Hummus with Cucumbers and Chicken

Meal 3: Low-Carb Meal
    Recipe: Grilled Wild Salmon with Quinoa and Edamame Salad

Meal 4: Low-Carb Meal
    Recipe: Chocolate Peanut Butter Shake

Meal 5: Low-Carb Meal
    Recipe: Cauli Mash and Meatballs

No Metabolic Mission: Day off!

Day 13: Accelerator: 10 minutes (minimum)

Select any activity of your choosing, and keep your heart rate above 120 beats per minute (bpm) the entire time. Prescribed optional interval for maximum results: Dirty Two-Thirties (2:30 low intensity / 2:30 high intensity)

LESSON 13
TAKE RESPONSIBILITY

He that is good for making excuses is seldom good for anything else.

—Benjamin Franklin

WARNING: We're going to be your superfriends and give you some tough love here. However, it is only because we care and want the best for you.

The number one red flag we look for when determining when someone is ready for transformation is acting and thinking like a victim. We know that people who blame others for their current condition, pain, suffering, and disappointment are people who have not yet accepted responsibility for their own choices. When we detect that kind of thinking, we do not choose those people for the journey of transformation…because we simply cannot help them. A victim mentality is not capable of change.

If someone cannot take responsibility for their actions, it is impossible for them to reach a goal.

You can decide whether you want to be a victim or not. But know this at the outset: Once someone chooses to take responsibility for their actions, then they *can* change! Taking responsibility is huge and scary and makes you extremely vulnerable. It takes a ton of courage, but courage is what it takes to change your life! It means you are responsible for your failures, your bad days, and all those times that you lost weight and gained it back again.

We're not saying that you haven't suffered in the past. We're not saying that awful things didn't happen to you. We're not saying that you aren't struggling, or that you don't have a chaotic and unpredictable life right now. What we *are* saying is that the only way you can change your life forever is to take full responsibility for your actions.

Here is your wake-up call: You are in the driver's seat! You always have been. You aren't struggling with your weight because someone held a gun to your head and forced you to consume 5,000 calories a day. You CHOSE to eat what you ate…when you ate it! Don't feel bad about it—heck, we've made a lot of poor choices, too, that cost us! However, take responsibility for it, and you can take your life wherever you wish. You can declare your dreams and make them a reality. You can write down your goals and achieve them. But first you need to take responsibility and stop blaming others for what has or has not happened for you.

This concept is pretty simple. Life is unexpected and unfair. Anything and everything can and will happen. You will break bones, you will throw out your back, you will have marital issues or career problems. You will be put on a different medication that causes unwanted side effects. But one thing is for sure: Life won't shove 5,000 calories down your throat. Only you can choose to do that. If you don't take responsibility and call yourself out for doing it, you're only protecting your destructive behavior…and you will never, ever change. But once you own it and admit it, you take full control of your actions and destiny!

We're not singling you out here. Heck, we *all* fall into the victim mind-set. In fact, we both struggle with this on a daily basis. It is *hard* to take responsibility for your actions. It sucks to feel like you messed up sometimes. But we're all human, and we mess up. However, it requires a ton of courage to take responsibility. Everyone around you will likely recognize your bravery.

Jeff's Terrible, Wonderful Tuesday

Jeff and his daughter Juliana had returned home after the 90-day boot camp feeling confident and resolute about their eating and exercise routines. Michelle, Jeff's wife, was 100 percent on board and made changes to how she shopped, cooked, and prepared meals for the entire family. But when Jeff began reporting back his results to us, something was off. The numbers just didn't add up. When we asked Jeff if he was following through on his promises to meet his goals, he assured us he was. So what was happening? We decided to take things into our own hands by running some light surveillance on Jeff. We wanted to believe that he was telling us the truth, but we also knew that when people are in their old, comfortable home environments, it can be difficult to resist their triggers and old habits.

After a few days of checking up on Jeff, we found that he was not doing what he said he was going to do. Jeff was eating well, in large part thanks to Michelle's efforts. But he was barely exercising at all. He wouldn't show at the gym, and when he did go, he would only stay a few minutes then leave. If he wanted to continue to lose weight, then he had to move every day.

We confronted him. Sitting in his living room, we gently asked him how it was going for him being at home. He said everything was great. When we pressed him about the discrepancies in his numbers, he angrily insisted that he was doing everything he said he was. Clearly, he was upset that we were questioning his integrity. When we kept probing and asking him if that was true, he hesitated and then broke down.

"I was so embarrassed and felt so ashamed. Here I was, sitting in front of Chris and Heidi, who had given me so much and trusted me so much. And I was lying to them. In my mind, I had been making all sorts of excuses for why I was cutting my exercise short—I had bad knees, bad back, and I had work to do. You name it, I had an excuse for it. These excuses were all about me playing the victim—they were ways for me to deflect responsibility for my choices and my actions. Did I not want to succeed? No! I wanted to reach my goals! But it took Chris and Heidi confronting me to really understand how to take responsibility once and for all."

Who was hurt by Jeff skipping his exercise and lying about it? Jeff.

Our excuses are simply that: reflections of us not being ready to take responsibility. But in the end, this "terrible, wonderful Tuesday" was a wake-up call that worked. The confrontation with us enabled Jeff to confront not only his excuses, but the lies that lay beneath the excuses. He chose to use a "victim" excuse and say that he couldn't exercise because of his knees—when in his heart he knew that he could have easily worked around his injuries and done exercises that didn't bother his knees. Jeff saw how his not being truthful was getting in his own way. "Lying to myself was just a way of giving myself an out for not being successful. Talk about a vicious circle!"

Why was this moment such a turning point for Jeff? Because his backslide was triggered when he broke his promise one day at home, and didn't follow through on his exercise. Instead of confessing, reassessing, and recommitting (the most powerful formula for getting back on track that we will discuss in the next section), it was easier for his ego to place the blame on something else, so he didn't have to take responsibility. Once he started blaming everything and everyone else, it was hard to stop the backslide, until we stepped in and challenged him to be vulnerable and honest, and take full responsibility. That was Jeff's turning point. He changed his mind-set, which has in turn changed his life. Now Jeff will tell you that his knees and back feel absolutely amazing since he's lost the weight…and that he has never felt more proud of who he is as a father and contributor to his community. Jeff lost nearly 200 pounds in a year and is now coaching others through the journey of transformation!

Heidi Tip

Fighting through injuries is no easy battle. I've been there! Many of you most likely have been, too—whether the result of overtraining or a freak accident, injuries even as small as a strained muscle can make us feel threatened that our fitness levels will slip away. They tend to even become excuses why we can't go to the gym, or even better yet, why we have to eat more junk food.☺ Our health and happiness have become victim to this injury. I'm not pointing fingers. I've been there, too!!! But it doesn't have to be this way—injuries are NOT excuses. There are alternative exercises around any injury.

For other people, taking responsibility is a more subtle process, but it requires the same kind of honesty and looking in the mirror. Taking responsibility isn't easy—it's the hard part. It takes vulnerability and courage, and is the true opportunity for growth and change. As we like to say, for every pointed finger, there are three pointing back! Ultimately, you didn't "end up" where you are at—your path and choices have led you to the place you are at. Life may have been rough, but you chose what you put in your mouth.

Here is the harsh reality: There are things in life we *can* control, and things in life we can't. We hear all the time, "I *have* to lose this weight or I will die."

Well, the truth is, you don't *have* to do anything. No one is holding a gun to your head…except you. If you choose to lose the weight, it is never because you *have* to. Always remember that it is because you *want* to!

Call to Action:
The Complain-and-Blame Exercise

1. List one to three times you attempted to lose weight and failed:

_____

_____

_____

_____

_____

_____

2. Now, explain why it didn't work:

_____

_____

_____

_____

_____

_____

3. Read over your responses and see if they contain either a complaint or a blame.

If you are placing the blame on anything or anyone other than yourself, then you are playing the victim—which will never lead to change.

What should the final response always be? The true one: "This diet didn't work because, regardless of the circumstances, I chose not to follow the program anymore."

We're not saying that something difficult or traumatic didn't happen to you. The reality of the situation is that somewhere on that time line, you *chose* not to follow the program anymore.

It's not easy to say, we know. However, this is what taking responsibility sounds like. Once you begin to think this way, you are ready for lifelong change!

Again, we say all of this out of love. Because thinking this way changed *our* lives for the better, changed our *peeps'* lives for the better, and will change *your* life for the better!

DAY 14

It's Time to Weigh In

Weigh in first thing in the morning without eating or drinking. Remove as many articles of clothing as possible to get the cleanest weight.

Your current weight: _____.

At this time, feel free to take any other measurements as well and note them here: _____

Day 14: Reset Day

It's Reset Day! Make meals easy by cooking up our Clean Cheat recipes, or simply add 1,000 extra calories of foods you love to a normal high-carb day.

Meal 1: Chocolate Glazed Crepes
Meal 2: BBQ Chicken Pita Pizza
Meal 3: Muddy Buddies
Meal 4: Mac and Cheese with Bacon
Meal 5: Homemade Oreos

Rest Day

Now relax! Take the day off and rest—no Metabolic Missions and no Accelerators!

LESSON 14:
CONQUER YOUR F.E.A.R.

Fear does not prevent death, it prevents living.

—Anonymous

Change is scary. We get it. Let's get it all out of the way right now:

You're scared of feeling deprived.

You're scared of the inconvenience of taking on new habits and patterns.

You're scared of feeling uncomfortable during the exercise.

You're scared of calling attention to your weight and don't want others to see or know that you're trying to do something about it.

You're scared of failing yet one more time at weight loss.

This is natural. This is normal. Fears are triggered when we explore out of our comfort zones. At the least sign of discomfort, we often automatically experience fear.

It's Just a Mirage

But what is FEAR? It's not tangible. It's not in the present, but in the future. FEAR is something that hasn't even happened. So what are you scared of?

To break it down, fear is not real. It's a reflection of what is in our imagination. Here's how we tear it apart.

Here's the most popular acronym for FEAR, and without a doubt the most appropriate one:

F—False

E—Evidence

A—Appearing

R—Real

False Evidence Appearing Real. Basically it's something untrue; it hasn't even happened, pretending to be real. Yet, we experience a physical reaction to it as if it were real.

Sounds easy. Maybe. We all have fears. We fear heights. We fear facing traumatic moments in our life. We fear feeling uncomfortable during exercise. We fear for our children's safety. We fear for our own health. We fear for each other's health. Believe it or not, many fear success, and the responsibility that comes along with it.

There are many things we FEAR—some consciously, some subconsciously. These are some common fears we hear from our peeps:

"I'm scared I won't be able to live happily without bingeing."

"I'm scared that I'm going to fail on yet *another* diet."

"I'm scared that if I mess this up, my family and friends are going to think I'm an even bigger disappointment."

"I'm afraid that if I start to exercise I'm going to have a heart attack."

"I'm scared of hurting my knee even more if I start exercising."

"I'm scared that if I commit to this, I will never get to eat my ice cream again."

"I'm scared of having to push myself physically."

"I'm scared of losing my friends by doing this."

Right now, think what it is about these fears that *actually* scares you. You're scared of something that hasn't happened...and here's the punchline: Chances are, it might not!

Now, think of all the things that these FEARs have *cost* you. They have cost you your dreams and opportunities at your ideal weight. They have cost you joy. They have cost you integrity. They have cost you confidence, self-esteem, and dignity.

In this guide, we share with you all of the tips and tactics to prevent nearly every one of these scenarios. Thing is, most of what we are scared of isn't life threatening or true, yet we let it completely paralyze us. We allow fear to hold us back from our true potential and greatness. Unfortunately, until we confront this "scary monster" of false evidence in front of us, we will never fulfill our dreams.

Mitzi had been chosen to be on the show, but we didn't realize the extent of Mitzi's misery and pain. She was over 100 pounds overweight—that's what we saw. What we didn't see was hidden inside of her home: She'd become a hoarder. Her home was in shambles. She had no refrigerator, no stove, no heat, nothing. It's not that she didn't have the money to fix it. She was so terrified of a repairman coming to the house and thinking poorly of her after seeing her living situation, she couldn't bring herself to ever call for help.

She was so scared of what other people would think of her, it was costing her a better quality of life. She was living in shame and embarrassment.

Like Mitzi, when you confront your fears, something magical will happen. When we stop running away from them, and begin running toward them, they almost always disappear! Most often, what we are terrified of happening, never does. In fact, the outcome is usually more favorable than we ever expected!

For Mitzi, when she returned home from boot camp—with her Transformation Team by her side—she confronted her FEAR. She rallied her community to help clean out her house. They came out in force, acknowledging and complimenting her bravery for opening up and being vulnerable. Sure enough, that incredible day she even made new friends and some of the best supporters on her Transformation Team! Mitzi literally emptied her house and rid herself of the sad, scared person she had become. She confronted the FEAR that had kept her imprisoned for years, and now has completely liberated herself!

Mitzi's greatest fear was admitting to herself—and the world—that she was a hoarder. Georgeanna's biggest fear was that her husband and kids wouldn't need her anymore if she put herself first. Bruce's biggest fear was that he wasn't worthy of love.

You are not alone. We all have FEARs and we will all continue to have fears throughout the rest of our lives. But now you have the opportunity to resee FEAR and see each fear you harbor inside as an opportunity for growth.

When you begin to "see" FEAR as life's opportunities for growth and strength, it takes all power away from those feelings and situations that scare you, and puts you in the driver's seat.

Try this exercise.

Call to Action: Letting Go of FEAR

1. What are you afraid of? Make a list. Most fears fall into one of four buckets:

   Fear of failure

   Fear of losing control

   Fear of losing connection/of rejection

   Fear of injury/discomfort/death

2. Now how do you respond to that fear?

   Do you sabotage your progress?

   Do you make excuses to quit or run away?

   Do you get angry or blame someone else?

   Do you withdraw into yourself so no one would know?

3. Okay. Now let's figure out what that fear is costing you.

   Have you lost love?

   Have you missed out on success?

   Have you disconnected from people you care about and who care about you?

   Have you broken a promise to yourself and lost integrity?

4. Next, what would it look like if you were to confront that fear? Stop with the False Evidence in your head—what is the *real* probable outcome?

The more you seek out these fears, identify what they are costing you, and then face them head-on, the more you will see them begin to shrivel and disappear.

Anytime you sense a fear cropping up, repeat the steps above.

Soon you will understand and feel that when you take on your fears and build trust in yourself, you can control them, and your life becomes limitless. Therein lies a path that is uniquely yours. Look at what you are capable of! And deep down inside, you know it. Look what FEAR has cost you. Not anymore!

Heidi Tip
Get Out of Your Comfort Zone!

One of my most popular blog posts from about a year ago was called "Once I Try, I'll Realize I CAN!" It was all about how hard it feels to get out of our comfort zone and try new things, which is a huge part of confronting our FEAR. Chris and I spend our lives challenging others to step outside their comfort zones to achieve a level of living that they've never before experienced. I think it's time I take my own advice and do the same. People so often think that because we help others accomplish great things, Chris and I have no fear in doing these things ourselves. I am here to correct those individuals. We *do* get scared! We *do* need people to push us to jump outside our comfort zones! Who does this for us? None other than… our show participants. ☺

When I wrote this post, I was spending time in New Zealand with one person in particular who reminds me how important it is to live my own life the way that I am teaching her to live. Melissa, because of you, I am spending this year being *UNcomfortable.* ☺ Like you have made it your mantra, I am making mine the same: I'm replacing "I can't" with "I'll try." **Once I try, I'll realize I CAN!**

POWELL

LIVE IT!

You have bravely dug deep over the past seven days, and have begun to remove some of the major roadblocks that have kept you from achieving your lifelong goals. From this place of newfound strength and clarity, you are now ready to take all of the incredible work you accomplished in the first 14 lessons, and build upon this new foundation for transformation you are creating. In the next seven days, we will coach you through *another radical shift in thinking* so that you have the know-how to live a life of transformation forever.

These lessons show you how to make concrete changes in your behavior. We will teach you the secret to never failing, how to balance your priorities, and give you a full forecast of what to expect on the journey ahead. We are going to show you how to zero in on the bad habits that have been sabotaging your weight loss and transform them into healthy, sustainable habits that will fuel your weight loss and fitness.

These are the final seven days and lessons to live a life of transformation. Take them in, embrace them, and hang on for the ride. Here we go!

DAY 15

Day 15: High-Carb Day

Meal 1: Breakfast
   Recipe: Power Mocha Shake with Fruit

Meal 2: High-Carb Meal
   Recipe: Strawberry and Banana Quinoa Muffins

Meal 3: High-Carb Meal
   Recipe: Turkey Sliders with Sweet Potato "Bun"

Meal 4: High-Carb Meal
   Recipe: Apple and Dip

Meal 5: Low-Carb Meal
   Recipe: Eggplant Curry Stir-Fry

Day 15: Metabolic Mission: The Countdown (Stepladder)

Set a running clock and, as fast as you can, do 21 reps of each exercise in the circuit, then 18 reps, then 15 reps, then 12, 9, 6, and 3.

Push-Ups
Hollow Rocks
Air Squats

Day 15: Accelerator: 15 minutes (minimum)

Select any activity of your choosing, and keep your heart rate above 120 beats per minute (bpm) the entire time. Prescribed optional interval for maximum results: Thrilling Thirties (:30 low intensity / :30 high intensity)

LESSON 15
GO ALL IN

If you always do what you've always done, you'll always get what you've always gotten.

—Tony Robbins

When Cassie started her journey of transformation, she would never go all in. She would report following "most" of the program, but always reserved reasons why she needed to do her own portions, make her own food choices, and follow advice contrary to the advice we gave her. She would justify her behavior by saying that she was the only one who truly understood her body and how it worked—but in reality she was just protecting her food addiction and wanted the option to binge when she wanted. Most important, she was too terrified to lose control. She had always held the power, control, keys to her life. By giving them up and going all in, she would need to admit that her way didn't work. Because of this, her weight kept stalling out. By the 90-day mark she was struggling to lose a pound a week. She finally came to terms with the fact that "Cassie's way doesn't work." "When I realized that I was no longer moving toward my goal weight, I realized I had to submit to the process that Chris and Heidi laid out for me—the one that had worked for so many people."

If Cassie was going to make a lifelong change, she had to give up what we call her "ace in the pocket" and follow the program that *does* work. So she went all in. And became one of our greatest transformations of all time.

Submitting to the process is a crucial step in your transformation journey. It's not just submitting to the diet and the exercise, it is acting upon *all* the lessons of transformation! This is the step that led to Cassie's huge success and her final accomplishment: not only the loss of 176 pounds, the rejuvenation of her marriage, and being reunited with her son, but most important, loving herself for the first time in decades.

Trust the Process

What do we mean by *trust the process*? We mean giving up that ace in your pocket, that "control card" that you hold on to, and throw down on the table to justify breaking your commitment to the plan. The mental conversation that we have is: "My body is different. I know and understand it better than anyone else, so I'll just do what works for me." Or it can also be based on a physical or emotional setback, such as "Well, they don't have a bad knee," or "They aren't dealing with the struggles that I have right now."

Trust us, we've heard it a million times before. This is the ultimate excuse, the reason of all reasons that your ego makes you feel like you are in control, because it is too afraid to show weakness or struggle. But deep down, you know you are simply protecting your bad behavior. Cassie spent so much time trying to convince herself that she knew her body better than anyone else. But she was lying to herself: Her body was *not* different. She, like all of us, abides by the laws of physics. The reality was that she did not have control over her binge eating.

Listen up: There are over 7 billion of us on this earth, and *all* of our bodies abide by the laws of physics, which dictate that if we take in less energy than we consume, we lose weight. If your body does not lose weight when at a calorie deficit, then your body defies the laws of physics. You need to put down this book and immediately check yourself in to a scientific research facility for evaluation.

Many people who struggle to lose weight and keep it off are struggling with something much larger than themselves: an unhealthy relationship with food and weight. Just take Heidi. For years as a teenager and young woman, she struggled with an eating disorder. "Although I am recovered, I still am vulnerable to the kind of thinking and behaviors that triggered my eating disorder to begin with."

And that's true for many people, Cassie included. When she was able to see that she was not in control of her food, she was able to see with clarity that she was simply a food addict. That revelation was ultimately liberating.

When you act like you don't have a problem, always justifying that your conditions in life are different, or your body is different than everyone else's, be aware that you are most likely hiding that ace in your back pocket!

Call to Action

What have you always used as the reason to never commit fully to other programs? What's your "ace in the pocket"? _____

_____

DAY 16

Day 16: High-Carb Day

Meal 1: Breakfast
  Recipe: Turkey Frittata

Meal 2: High-Carb Meal
  Recipe: Sweet Wrap

Meal 3: High-Carb Meal
  Recipe: Barbecue Chicken Salad

Meal 4: High-Carb Meal
  Recipe: Peanut Butter Shake

Meal 5: Low-Carb Meal
  Recipe: Curry Turkey Sliders with Cucumber and Tomato Salad

Day 16: Metabolic Mission: Afterburner (Rounds for Time)

Set a running clock and do 5 rounds of the following exercises as fast as you can, but keeping good form!

20 Back Lunges
15 Push-Ups

Day 16: Accelerator: 15 minutes (minimum)

Select any activity of your choosing, and keep your heart rate above 120 beats per minute (bpm) the entire time. Prescribed optional interval for maximum results: Tenacious Twos (2:00 low intensity / 2:00 high intensity)

LESSON 16
FALL WITHOUT FAILING

> *Our greatest glory consists not in never falling, but in rising every time we fall.*
>
> —Oliver Goldsmith

Sometimes the unexpected happens. And even though you now know how your promises are the most important thing in the world, sometimes you're just not going to keep one. This is to be expected.

Let's face it: You're human. We all make mistakes. You're going to mess up and break promises along the journey. You're going to eat what you shouldn't. You're going to skip a workout...or two. You're going to have some bad days. You're going to fall flat on your face when you least expect it.

This sounds awful, doesn't it? Because in your past, falling flat on your face meant that you'd failed yet again. Meant less self-love, less trust and belief in yourself.

Well, we have good news for you. *Falling* no longer needs to mean *failing*.

When you commit to Extreme Transformation, you are embracing a path where it's impossible to fail.

How so?

We know the secret lifeline to prevent failing.

Built into Extreme Transformation is the proven formula for getting back on your feet and continuing your journey. It is the lifeline you will *always* have the choice to grab onto when you fall. This is one of the most powerful shifts in your thinking during your journey of transformation. It is inevitable that you will mess up sometime. When you do, the backslide will begin. To stop the bleeding, and get back on your feet, you must learn and *apply* this formula:

Confess + Reassess + Recommit

These three simple actions, when done in this order, have a profound impact. This will be one of the most valuable lessons you can learn on the journey, and you will use it time and again!

Call to Action

1. **Have the courage to confess.** If you made a mistake, fell off the wagon, or just didn't keep a promise in one way or another, you have to admit it. Trust us, this is easier said than done. If you ask *anyone* who has been through the journey of transformation, they will tell you that this is one of the most difficult parts. It takes us right back to the very first and most important step: Be vulnerable. It takes a ton of courage to admit to others our imperfections, but until you do, the weight of the broken promise will hold you back. Walk right over to the nearest mirror, look yourself in the eye, and say out loud the promise you broke to yourself. When you are ready, find someone on your trusted Transformation Team, or your superfriend, and tell them about your slip-up and that you need to confess what happened. Don't hold back and be vague—it will not be a full confession and it will hold you back. Share the details and get it *all* off of your shoulders. Confessing takes resolve and courage, but it also gives you a new sense of energy and trust in yourself. You can't look back.

   There are two dangerous reasons why most people don't confess, and eventually fail:

1. You are protecting your destructive habits and *want* to fall off the program to eat poorly again.

2. You are using negative self-talk and telling yourself that you don't want to be a burden to your Transformation Team or superfriend. This is a lie to yourself. Your team wants to see you succeed. It doesn't matter if you need to confess every week, or even every other day. Reach out to them!

2. Reassess the promise or promises that you have made and the goals that you fell short of. Ask yourself: *Why did I break that promise?* Was the commitment unattainable in your busy life and too hard to keep? Or was it a fluke day when things happened that were out of your control and you simply ran out of time? Were you feeling lonely, anxious, or stressed about something in your life? For most people, reassessing a mistake or setback reveals one of three things:

- An emotional trigger that overpowered your promise.
- An old excuse based upon the old you.
- Your promise is too far out of reach of your current position and is therefore not realistic or attainable now.

Reassessing your transformation vision clarifies what's possible for you right now. You need to go back to your goals and see if they are SMART.

Ask yourself if your goal is:

- Specific
- Measurable
- Attainable
- Relevant
- Time-bound

Without our realizing it, most of our slip-ups happen because our goals become imprecise or unrealistic. Take a good look at the circumstances and decide whether to continue with the same commitment, or if you should reduce it to something that you *know* you can keep.

3. Rise up and recommit: Once you have reassessed and feel unbelievably confident that you can keep your new commitment, it is time to recommit to your promises and your goals. Contact someone on your team and declare your recommitment. Say it loud and say it clear!

Reassessing your promise and your goals makes it possible to know exactly where you are right now in your journey and what is realistic to expect from yourself. When you go through the process of establishing promises that are truly SMART, then you will not be afraid to move on after a setback. You will also feel more determined and confident that you can indeed keep that promise and reach that goal. When you stand up and once again declare your promises and goals, you strengthen your commitment to yourself!

Merhbod had lost over 100 pounds in just six months and was well on his way to his ideal weight. Then slowly but surely his weight loss slowed to a stop...and he began to gain it all back. We had no idea because he kept sending weigh-in pictures and video showing that he was continuing to lose weight, when in reality he was rigging his scale at home to make it look like he was. This went on for three months until Mehrbod finally realized that the addict had completely taken over. He was terrified to disappoint us, but he knew there was only one way to stop the backslide. He picked up the phone and called us. We met with him, and he confessed everything. We took it all in, and when he was finished he put his face in his hands and cried. We lifted his head, looked him in the eyes, and said, "Thank you. We can only imagine the courage it took to do that."

Immediately, we could see an emotional weight lifted off his shoulders. He sat back, took a deep breath, and said, "What can I do now?" We reassessed his goals and daily commitments, and when we came up with something totally attainable, he recommitted. Sure enough, he went on to break weight-loss records in the final three months of his transformation, and qualified for skin-removal surgery. When Merhbod summoned the courage to confess, reassess, and recommit, he broke free from the backslide, got back up on his feet, and surged forward with more vigor than ever before. We cannot underestimate the power of this formula.

As Lisa recalls, "I remember the first time I messed up a couple weeks into my transformation. I doubled my portions for dinner one night. Didn't seem like a big deal, but it haunted me, because deep down I knew I had broken a commitment to myself. I fell back into my old way of thinking and felt like I was a failure. Sure enough, I ended up overeating the next couple nights, until I remembered what Chris and Heidi taught me about falling without failing. I knew that if I didn't stop the bleeding, it was going to take me down, and I would fail yet again. It was so hard to pick up the phone and confess, but when I did I immediately felt control again. Together, we reassessed and recommitted. It was the lifeline I needed. I messed up a handful of times on my weight loss journey, and every time, I used this same formula—and it got me to my goal. Without a doubt, it was the greatest lesson I learned on the journey!"

As Jami described for us, "The 90-day boot camp was just the beginning of my transformation. The real work happened when I returned home. It took me a while to realize that the journey I was on was really the rest of my life. I had always lived my life in an all-or-nothing way. If I ever messed up, that was it. I was a failure and I'm done. Maybe a year later I'd try again. And that just set me up to fail—over and over again. Now I understand what Chris and Heidi mean when they say it's okay to fall—it's just an opportunity to get back up again. This way of thinking about mistakes is so much more realistic and encouraging than thinking of failure as a personal quality or source of shame. That's the old Jami. I just don't think that way anymore."

If you break a promise, will it start the downward spiral again? Will you once again give up on yourself, beat yourself up, and find yourself in a dark place?

Now you have the lifeline. You can *choose* the single most powerful and proven formula to get back on your feet, or you can *choose* to quit.

When you break a promise to yourself, it is not cause for shame or embarrassment. In fact, mistakes and setbacks are the training ground for flexing the real muscles of transformation—the muscles that get you back up on your feet and moving toward your goal. This is why during your transformation journey you will learn to fall...not fail. This is one of the key steps of your journey—learning how to clear broken promises, strategize an easier path toward your goal, and move forward with more enthusiasm than ever before.

The power is now in your hands. Any time you fall, you are always just three simple steps away from being right back on track.

Perfectly Imperfect

Disappointment happens when expectations are not met. Simple as that. Most people make the grave mistake of setting unrealistic expectations for themselves. They create a vision of perfection that not only is impossible to fulfill but also hampers their ability to stay on their journey. When these expectations are not met, the strong emotions tied with disappointment come flooding in. In these times, most people lose the magical ingredient of *belief* and any further effort (and progression) toward the goal comes to a rapid halt.

Remember: We are all *perfectly imperfect*. That's the awesome part about being human. It is working through our setbacks and slip-ups that creates our uniqueness and character. Why place such expectations of perfection on yourself when they are simply unrealistic? Without messing up, we could never appreciate the beauty that life offers us along the way.

Heidi Tip

I am perfect.

Perfectly imperfect, that is.

I use the word *perfect* a lot, and often people remind me that nothing is perfect. I totally disagree. I believe that everyone and everything is perfect and beautiful in its imperfect state of being. Think about that for one second—imagine that just maybe your imperfections actually make you perfect. Don't you just love the freedom that thought gives you? Well, time to realize the reality of the thought and let go of our self-judgments and negative self-talk. It's time to embrace our imperfections. Now, I'm not saying to throw caution to the wind and go indulge in a gallon of super-chunky triple chocolate fudgy goo. I'm saying that it's okay to mess up, and it's okay to have faults. For those of you who don't, I'm sorry. These faults, trials, imperfections, and stumbles are some of our greatest blessings—they're our springboard to becoming the strongest person we can possibly be!

XO Heidi

DAY 17

Day 17: High-Carb Day

Meal 1: Breakfast

    Recipe: Turkey and Potato Skillet Breakfast

Meal 2: High-Carb Meal

    Recipe: Strawberry and Banana Quinoa Muffins

Meal 3: High-Carb Meal

    Recipe: Italian Tuna and White Bean Lettuce Wraps

Meal 4: High-Carb Meal

    Recipe: Greek Yogurt Parfait with Fruit

Meal 5: Low-Carb Meal

    Recipe: Barbecue Grilled Pork Tenderloin

Day 17: Metabolic Mission: Chippin' Away (Chipper)

Set a running clock and see how long it takes you to do these exercises. Record your time in your Daily Tracker!

100 Jumping Jacks
75 Air Squats
50 Push-Ups
25 Kickbacks

Day 17: Accelerator: 15 minutes (minimum)

Select any activity of your choosing, and keep your heart rate above 120 beats per minute (bpm) the entire time. Prescribed optional interval for maximum results: Nasty Nineties (1:30 low intensity / 1:30 high intensity)

LESSON 17
BE BENEFICIALLY SELFISH

Make your own recovery the first priority in your life.

—Robin Norwood

The journey of transformation requires that you put yourself first. Plain and simple. If you don't put your needs, your promises, your goals first, then you will not succeed. For many (especially us parents), this can seem totally selfish. We are programmed to put our families first. However, this programming is actually a bit faulty. While our family may be the most important people in the world to us, if something happens to you that affects your ability to be a good parent, the family suffers in the long run. Nobody captured the importance of our own health better than the FAA and their safety guidelines for airplane emergency situations in the cabin.

We are ordered to put an oxygen mask over our own mouth before we turn to help a child or another person. For good reason: If you can't breathe, how can you help your child, your neighbor, and everyone else around you?

The same rule applies for your health.

If it isn't a "life-or-death" situation; Other people and their needs can wait. They can be uncomfortable for a moment while you ensure *your* health and survival—so that you can be there for them in the future.

We call this being *beneficially selfish*. Our society and culture have taught us that it is selfish to put ourselves before others. In actuality, we are taking care of ourselves first, *for the benefit of everyone around us.* Keep in mind that as you take this step and make this shift in thinking, others around you might still be programmed by society and culture, and many will likely call you "selfish" for putting yourself first. They just don't see the bigger picture. Explain it to them if you like, but either way, it is the truth.

Over time, putting everyone else's needs first pushes most people into dire health situations. Look at the position you are in right now, and what has led you here. Maybe you're frustrated with the 20 pounds that is taking forever to come off. Or perhaps you picked up this book after a triple bypass surgery. Either way, making yourself a priority in your life is of utmost importance— not just to your physical health, but to your mental and emotional health as well!

When we are fulfilling promises and taking care of ourselves, we feel better about ourselves and can bring more joy into the lives of our families and friends. How much joy did you spread when you felt like crap about yourself? Want to bring more long-term joy into the lives of everyone around you, your family, your friends, your children? Be beneficially selfish!

After years of putting her son first, Kathy declared independence so that she could finally take care of herself. David also had to learn how to put himself first. When he was working 14-hour days, he reduced his hours to 11 per day, to carve out time for his health. In fact, all the people you have met so far in this book have had to learn how to put themselves first and make their health and fitness journeys their number one priority.

For Georgeanna this lesson, this step in her transformation journey, was one of the most difficult to actualize. "I only saw myself as a pastor's wife who was meant to serve—serve God, my husband, my children, my community. I didn't even know how to take care of myself, never mind put myself first. But I did learn. And what I realized is that when you surround yourself with loving people who really do understand what you are trying to do, then you can put yourself first without guilt or looking over your shoulder."

Call to Action

In general we all have some predictable features of our lives, but their importance varies depending on our life and situation. Also, our priorities shift over the course of our lives. When we are young and don't yet have families to take care of, we might position education and social life over staying in touch with relatives. When we are older, education may not be as important and our health seems to shift in its importance.

When you think about your totem pole, rank these values based upon your present— where you are now, what you need now, and what your goals are now. Take a look at the following list and put these items in order, with the most important on top.

- Education
- Family
- Friends/social
- Religion
- Physical and Mental Health
- Serving others
- Work

Being beneficially selfish usually requires a sit-down meeting with your support system (and family and friends), to speak openly about your journey and priorities. Teach them what you just learned and that you are going to be putting yourself first in many situations, not because you are being generally selfish, but because you know that when you are healthy and fit, you can provide that much more to their lives. Talk openly about the journey ahead, and help them find solutions for things like transportation and meals, for when you are not available:

Reality Check

There will always be a valid reason why you should put someone/something else first. Once again, unless the situation is truly life or death (or a health scare), you know in your heart what you *should* do—take care of yourself first.

Chris Tip

It's necessary to have realistic expectations of life so that you are fully prepared. Here is a glimpse into your likely future. This is what you can expect from life over the course of your weight loss journey...and beyond:

- Loss and tragedy
- Family struggles
- Career struggles
- Financial struggles
- Relationship struggles
- Overall bad days

Events such as these are inevitable and unavoidable. Expect them to happen, because they will. It is our natural tendency to fall back into comforting habits, or put things on hold with our health so that we can handle such issues as those listed above. However, we are here to tell you that these are everyday occurrences in life. With many of these events ahead of you, there will never be a right time in the future to make your health and fitness a priority. The only right time...is right now.

If you play your cards right, you may have a good 75 to 100 total years here on earth. And not for one second will anyone walk in your shoes. This is *your* journey. Aggressively defend it. Do it for your health, for your happiness, and for the subsequent benefit of your family, friends, and loved ones. Let nothing get in the way of your destiny and what you deserve. Get your priorities straight!

DAY 18

Day 18: High-Carb Day

Meal 1: Breakfast
  Recipe: Pumpkin Spice Vanilla Protein Pancakes

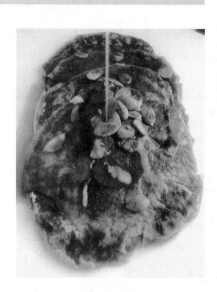

Meal 2: High-Carb Meal
  Recipe: Hulk Shake

Meal 3: High-Carb Meal
  Recipe: Loaded Potato

Meal 4: High-Carb Meal
  Recipe: PB & J Rice Cakes and Shake

Meal 5: Low-Carb Meal
  Recipe: Fajita Chicken Roll-Ups with Roasted Squash and Avocado Puree

Day 18: Metabolic Mission: "Go Time" (AMRAP)

Set a running clock and do as many rounds of the following circuit as you can in 11 minutes.

7 Push-Ups
9 Leg Levers
11 High Knees

Day 18: Accelerator: 15 minutes (minimum)

Select any activity of your choosing, and keep your heart rate above 120 beats per minute (bpm) the entire time. Prescribed optional interval for maximum results: Mighty Minutes (1:00 low intensity / 1:00 high intensity)

LESSON 18
HAVE REALISTIC EXPECTATIONS OF OTHERS

You're in the midst of a war: a battle between the limits of a crowd seeking the surrender of your dreams, and the power of your true vision to create and contribute. It is a fight between those who will tell you what you cannot do, and that part of you that knows, and has always known, that we are more than our environment; and that a dream, backed by an unrelenting will to attain it, is truly a reality with an imminent arrival.

—Tony Robbins

You may not want to hear this, but we are determined to be honest and up front with you: Your family and friends may not be your best supporters. As you begin to make changes in your life, the people around you may very well feel uncomfortable. Your changes affect their status quo. They may claim that they want to support you and that they want you to succeed at your goals. But often, they are really, really uncomfortable with how *your* changes make *them* feel.

We are by no means saying that your family and friends are bad or malicious, but chances are that your goals and new life may not work well with what they are used to. In fact, your new lifestyle can be downright threatening. Unless they understand and embrace change, most people wince with discomfort if asked to move out of their comfort zone. So as innocent humans not yet on their own journey of transformation, some of the people in your life might react negatively to your new choices and newfound confidence.

- When you start to eat healthy, stop drinking, and spend more time at the gym, your boyfriend or wife may feel abandoned.
- When you stop indulging in pizza and wings, and instead choose healthier options every three hours, your buddy might feel angry that you've ditched him and your shared Friday-night routine.
- When you make your health a priority, your children or spouse might feel jealous of lost time and express resentment.

Everyone has a reaction. But it's up to you to surround yourself with those who understand and truly support your journey and perhaps distance yourself from those, including family, who might be trying to impede your success. Now, we are not saying that you should distance yourself from your friends, family, and loved ones simply because they may express some frustration with the process.

But by having realistic expectations of their responses to you, you will not get distracted or disappointed. You can separate your goals from *their* desires and practice patience and perseverance (and compassion for them) even in the face of adversity! There is a very good chance that your friends and family *do* love and support you…chances are, they are just terrified of losing you in their life. it's just nearly impossible for them to understand what you are going through since they are not walking in your shoes.

What's the best response? *Love!* Even if friends or family try to pull you from the process or get upset with your new routines that might be causing them an inconvenience, you can think and respond to them in love—*as long as* doing so doesn't compromise your own goals.

Part of this loving response is learning how to communicate effectively with those you care about. If the way your friend/family is being is pulling you away from your goals, you should feel confident enough to pull them aside and have a loving, open communication about what your goals are, and what you need from them (support) to get there. Express to them that you know they love you, and that is why you feel safe having this conversation.

For instance, you might say, "I know you don't think you are hurting me when you try to get me to eat dessert with the family, but it triggers an impulse in me to binge that I can't control. Please don't take it personally when I decline your homemade ice cream...I love you no less, but need to focus on my health."

As you make changes in how you eat, how you live, and the choices you make, you will likely trigger discomfort in your friends, family, and co-workers. Changing your routine, the way you eat, and when you're available impacts all those with whom you regularly come in contact. Many of our peeps tell us they seem to have "lost" their friends or even family members. You might hear words from them like "You've abandoned us" and "You think you're too good for us now."

You might also hear people begin to doubt you, question you, even criticize you. When one person changes, everyone around that person is affected. Sometimes this reaction will stem from a sort of jealousy—they are struggling with seeing your success while they are stuck in their unhappy life. The best thing to do is to love your friends and family regardless and lead by example.

But remember: If you aren't getting the love or support you need, you should expand (not replace) your circle of friends and supporters and include more people who are more aligned with your vision and goals. These people are most likely members of your gym, running group, or support team. As Dr. Holly says, "A connection to others who are living a similar lifestyle improves the odds of success." Which is why it's so important to look again at your social connections.

Mitzi felt that she didn't quite lose the people in her life, but rather that those who didn't understand or support all the changes she was making simply drifted away. "I didn't feel any ill will—it has just been a case of being in different places. And you know what? It's all right. It doesn't necessarily mean that our two roads won't ever converge again."

Mitzi points out something important: *It's all right.* It's all right if people don't seem to like the new you. It's all right to lose touch with a friend or family member. It's all right because you are learning to put yourself first. When you live your life with you as the number one priority, you will begin to feel so much more at ease with your choices. You will feel clear and confident, instead of tangled up in trying to please other people.

1. Be beneficially selfish. You can't help anyone else if you can't help yourself first! Expect some to be upset and withdraw. This is an example of conditional love. In this journey toward loving ourselves, we need unconditional love and support.

2. Schedule time for *you* to fulfill your commitments, and time for *them*. They might give you a hard time, but if you communicate what is important and necessary to you and your health, then you have done everything in your power to keep communication open in the relationship.

There will always be reasons not to follow what you know in your heart is the path toward your health and happiness. Sometimes you have to go out of your way to get there. Honor your word over your reasons, and you will get there.

It is your time. Now go get 'em!

Chris & Heidi

DAY 19

Day 19: Low-Carb Day

Meal 1: Breakfast
   Recipe: No-Bake Oats

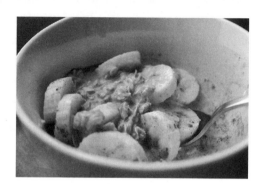

Meal 2: Low-Carb Meal
   Recipe: Quinoa Bites with
Zucchini, Tomato, and Arugula

Meal 3: Low-Carb Meal
   Recipe: Citrus Salmon Slaw

Meal 4: Low-Carb Meal
   Recipe: Popeye Shake

Meal 5: Low-Carb Meal
   Recipe: Chipotle Turkey Burger with House Pickles

Day 19: Metabolic Mission: Wake-Up Call (Tabata)

For each exercise, do as many reps as you can in 20 seconds. Rest for 10 seconds, then do as many reps as you can in 20 seconds again. Repeat for 8 total rounds (for a total of 4 minutes) per exercise. The lowest number of reps you get in any round is your score. You'll get one score per exercise. Add up all three scores, and record it in your Daily Tracker!

Kickbacks
Leg Levers
Air Squats

Day 19: Accelerator: 15 minutes (minimum)

Select any activity of your choosing, and keep your heart rate above 120 beats per minute (bpm) the entire time. Prescribed optional interval for maximum results: Dirty Two-Thirties (2:30 low intensity / 2:30 high intensity)

LESSON 19
REPLACE YOUR ADDICTION

Nothing tastes as good as being skinny feels.

—Anonymous

In transformation, we use the word *addiction* because it is a very powerful way to describe the impact of our habits. You may be a true food addict and engage in compulsive behavior, or you may simply have a bad series of habits that led to weight gain. Either way, the fact remains that in order for a new habit to be effective, the payoff *must be* more desirable than the habit you are replacing it with. This is true of relationships with food and other addictive substances.

As you have moved through the lessons of transformation, we have pointed out places and times when it's necessary to change your behavior in order to stay committed to your new lifestyle. Essentially, what we have been asking you to do is replace your addiction to junk food or soda, with eating foods that don't create such a strong physical craving. If you don't replace the addiction, it will simply reassert its control over you. For example, we understand that junk food is both positively reinforcing and rewarding—it acts upon the reward pathways of the brain and triggers you to want to repeat the behavior—but when done repeatedly over time, it comes with a heavy cost to your appearance and health. You get fat and sick.

When it comes to the weight loss journey, we are asking you to replace the satisfaction and enjoyment of eating what you want, when you want, and living a sedentary life with little to no exercise—with eating structured meals, eating on a schedule, and moving on a daily basis.

When looking at the two lifestyles, the former is more attractive. Of course everybody wants to eat whatever they want, whenever they want! However, that lifestyle comes at a great cost. When you look at the beneficial outcome of the latter, it quickly becomes the frontrunner!

What Is an Addiction?

Addiction is a state characterized by compulsive engagement in rewarding stimuli, despite adverse consequences. The two properties that characterize all addictive stimuli are that they are (positively) reinforcing (they increase the likelihood that a person will seek repeated exposure to them) and intrinsically rewarding (they activate the brain's "reward pathways" and are therefore perceived as being something positive or desirable).

The Payoff of Your New Habits

Everything has a cost and a payoff. The major cost of your new lifestyle is no longer having the convenience of eating what you want, when you want. Instead, you eat new foods that don't have the same reward impact, but keep you full for a long period of time. You can indulge, but only when it is customized into your plan and still accommodates your weight loss. As you are on the journey of transformation, here are some of the new payoffs you are now receiving:

- You are losing weight on the scale every week—and you feel good.
- Your clothes are looser—you may just need to invest in a new wardrobe!
- You are healthier.
- You are more attractive.

- You are seeing your body develop shapely muscles.
- You are getting an endorphin rush and euphoric sense of well-being from the exercise.
- You have a sense of pride, accomplishment, and control over your life.
- You are receiving accolades and respect from others—we are certain that you are the happy recipient of compliments and well-deserved praise.

All of the above results are payoffs for your new lifestyle. These payoffs are positively reinforcing. They do not always play directly upon the reward pathways of the brain in an immediate sense, but they do offer long-term fulfillment. The question is: Are the payoffs to your transformation more rewarding than the immediate satisfaction from food?

The purpose of this lesson is to create an awareness of the trade-offs that have happened here: what you have given up with your old life, for what you are getting with your new life. Granted, your new life is much more attractive (literally), but we want you to begin thinking ahead to when you reach your goal and some of these payoffs don't occur as often. Enjoy the payoffs of the weight loss journey now, but we will explore in much more detail the process of finding another new addiction as you transition from weight loss into maintenance.

Your New Addiction

When you hit your goal or are near your goal weight, some of the most powerful payoffs from the weight loss journey go away. While you once looked forward to seeing the number on the scale drop every week, it begins to remain more constant. While you beamed from the positive comments and pats on the back from your family and friends, they are all accustomed to you looking this way now, and may even become critical of your appearance again.

When the compliments stop coming, we begin to look for payoffs again. Our old habits and food addictions can creep back in. As humans we *need* something to satisfy our reward pathways. We need something to look forward to daily. When this weight loss phase is over, if you don't have a *new* addiction, you will quickly turn back to food, and begin to gain weight again.

So what will your new addiction be? See chapter 4.

DAY 20

Day 20: Low-Carb Day

Meal 1: Breakfast
   Recipe: Breakfast Frittata Veggie "Muffins"

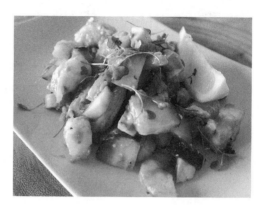

Meal 2: Low-Carb Meal
   Recipe: Protein Punch Wraps

Meal 3: Low-Carb Meal
   Recipe: Grilled Lamb Kebabs

Meal 4: Low-Carb Meal
   Recipe: Shrimp Cocktail Salad

Meal 5: Low-Carb Meal
   Recipe: Creamy Cauliflower Soup

No Metabolic Mission: Day Off!

Day 20: Accelerator: 15 minutes (minimum)

Select any activity of your choosing, and keep your heart rate above 120 beats per minute (bpm) the entire time. Prescribed optional interval for maximum results: Thrilling Thirties (:30 low intensity / :30 high intensity)

LESSON 20
TRIGGERS AND TACTICS

God, grant me the serenity to accept the things I cannot change, the courage to change the things I can, and the wisdom to know the difference.

—Serenity Prayer

We are surrounded by triggers all day, every day. The people in our lives, the places we pass through, the rituals of our daily routines. These triggers can evoke an emotional response in us. Some can be stronger than others, but either way any reaction can influence our decision-making ability.

When we encounter strong triggers, powerful emotions surface—so strong that we feel the need to soothe or numb ourselves when the emotion is negative, or to heighten the euphoria when the emotion is positive. We look outside ourselves for an instant comfort or way to make the high last longer. Unfortunately what we reach for can often set off a domino effect of old habits and behaviors, such as eating a pint of ice cream or racing over to the nearest convenience store for a package of donuts or a case of beer.

This lesson is all about being clear on your triggers—those situations, behaviors, and surroundings that tempt you to go back to your old ways. The beauty is this: Once you identify your *triggers*, you can see them more clearly. You can also train yourself to avoid them and resist them by using *tactics* that support you and your journey.

Just like habits, triggers can take time to dissipate. The purpose of a tactic is not to make the trigger go away, but to distract or empower the mind to prevent the emotional response. Most triggers can last for 5 to 15 minutes, so rest assured that if you employ these tactics to keep your mind and emotions occupied, you *can* navigate easily around or through any trigger!

People Triggers

Oddly enough, people triggers don't have as much to do with the actual person triggering you; people triggers are more about ourselves. People triggers usually stem from a deep emotional need that we feel is not being met. For example, our parent, teacher, boss, or partner might trigger within us:

- The need to feel loved
- The need to feel trusted
- The need to feel valued
- The need to feel desired
- The need to be respected
- The need to be right
- The need to be understood
- The need for freedom
- The need to be in control

This list just scratches the surface. We have many more emotional needs that might trigger us. We become reliant on one or more of these needs because at some point in our life, that basic emotional need worked to benefit us in some way. So we learned that when that emotional need is fulfilled, the results are typically positive. However, when we feel that the need is not being met, the reaction is usually one of anger or fear—both powerful triggers that turn many of us to junk food to numb and cope.

Tactics for People Triggers

1. Write down one to three emotional needs that you have:

   1. _____
   2. _____
   3. _____

2. Do your own reality check: Is this person really denying you of your emotional need, or preventing you from getting it? Does this person have enough relevance in your life that they have this power over you?

3. If they do hold enough relevance in your life, and you feel it is important that you receive the emotional need from this person, try communicating it with them. Let them know how you feel and how important it is to be trusted, valued, et cetera.

4. If you find yourself emotionally charged and it is clear that this individual will not help satisfy your emotional need, then it is time to separate yourself from this situation:
   - Relax and shift your focus to your breathing.
   - Choose one word that describes how you want to be in this moment: calm, relaxed, powerful, centered, or the like.
   - Reach out to a member of your Transformation Team to help you sort through your reaction to the person or situation that is triggering you.

Food Triggers

As humans, we are programmed from infancy for food to be soothing and comforting for us. We develop an emotional connection with sweet and savory comfort foods, overloaded with sugar, salt, and fat. These "hyperpalatables" release the feel-good endorphins in our brains. Because of this, such food helps to calm and relax us when we experience feelings of anger, sadness, anxiety, or loneliness. It will even heighten feelings of happiness. It's no surprise that these hyperpalatables have become one of the biggest addictions in the United States and abroad. Because they act on many of the same systems of the brain as many drugs, these comfort foods have become an emotional "painkiller" for the masses.

It doesn't help that we are also bombarded by junk food advertisements on TV, online, in newspapers, magazines—all over our media.

Tactics for Food Triggers

If you find that certain foods trigger binge behavior, use these tactics to beat the binge:

1. Use teamwork. Call or text someone on your Transformation Team to talk about how you are feeling. Simply talking about the issue is one of the most powerful steps in creating awareness and taking control of the trigger.

2. Clean out your environment of any trigger foods (you should have done that in Lesson 4!).

3. Avoid places, restaurants, or situations where you might find your trigger foods (the break room at work, drive-thru row, your friend's house that's loaded with junk food). Those who've successfully transformed themselves sometimes actually found alternative routes to get where they needed to go, just to avoid these dangerous pitfalls.

4. Have healthy options available at any moment: fruit, nuts, protein bars, protein shakes, gum, flavored water, and so on. Whatever you need to satisfy a sweet or salty craving, there are hundreds of amazing healthy alternatives available!

5. Stay on track with your five meals a day. Skipping a meal or snack will put you in low blood sugar, a vulnerable place for a trigger!

Event Triggers

Some of the main triggers we experience on a regular basis are event triggers. These powerful triggers are made up of a multitude of situational events such as going to a restaurant, social gathering, party, or family reunion. Even going to work can be a trigger for some people. The drive to and from work, walking by the break room or cafeteria, finally getting the kids to bed and sitting down on the couch—these regular daily events can trigger responses in us that make us want to reach for food.

Boredom is actually one of the biggest event triggers we can experience. You know, those moments in the middle of the day when the kids are at school and the spouse is at work...and you find yourself wandering aimlessly around the kitchen pantry. Or when you have hours to kill doing xyz...

Believe it or not, another huge event trigger for some can be finishing a long workout. Many people feel the need to reward themselves after a good sweat session and then develop a food reward habit that negates all of their hard work!

Whatever habits have been formed during these daily events can be difficult to break. One of our peeps confessed to us that the simple click of his seat belt always triggered a craving for fast food because for years, nearly every time he got into a car he would hit a drive-thru wherever he was going.

Certain times of the year are loaded with powerful triggers—our birthdays, the holidays, the anniversary of a breakup. When we are reminded of certain powerful events in our lives, our triggers can be summoned.

We have created a list of tactics that can help guide you through the toughest of event triggers. Find the triggers and tactics that best apply to your life!

Tactics for Going to a Restaurant

1. Eat something healthy before you go out and just order something extremely light when you are there.
2. Order an appetizer or side order instead of an entrée.
3. Order an entrée and cut it in half as soon as it is served. Eat half, and take the rest to go.
4. Ask your server to remove or not serve any trigger food items beforehand (say, chips, bread, soup or salad before the meal).
5. Choose a dish that has been steamed, baked, or grilled instead of fried or sautéed.

Tactics for the Drive to and from Work

1. Avoidance. Choose a different route to and from work so you don't pass by your drive-thru trigger.
2. Be prepared. Eat something before you leave home and before you leave work. If you are hungry on your drive, your inner voice will create any excuse it can to rationalize your destructive habit. *Do not break your promise!*
3. Keep your "why" in front of you. Keep a picture on your dashboard in the car. Never forget why you are doing this and how much better your life is going to be!

Tactics for Social Gatherings

1. Eat before you arrive.
2. Avoid the areas with food.
3. Chew gum.

4. Get a glass of water, soda water, or diet soda and keep it in your hands the whole time. We call this "glassing." It keeps your hands occupied and prevents you from feeling out of place.

Tactics for Workplace Triggers

1. Avoid the trigger areas as much as possible. If necessary, find alternative routes around the break room, cafeteria, vending machine, and so on.
2. Keep your desk well stocked with healthy options at all times.
3. Rally your co-workers to join the health and fitness bandwagon. This has become extremely popular these days, with thousands of businesses now offering only healthy options in their break rooms, cafeterias, and vending machines.

Tactics for End-of-Day Triggers

Typically after a long and stressful day, we feel the deep-rooted need to reward ourselves. Walking in the door from work, getting the kids to bed, or typing up those final emails can trigger some monster cravings for something that will derail you. Here's what to do:

1. Keep your hands and taste buds busy. Chew gum. Have your flavored water or low-calorie beverage in hand.
2. Grab the chopped veggies. They will give you a nice crunchy snack and fill you up.
3. Go to bed. We call the time from around 7:00 p.m. until you go to bed the "red zone." This is typically the time of the day when people are most likely to succumb to triggers and cravings. Ben Franklin said it best: "Early to bed, early to rise, makes a man healthy, wealthy, and wise."

Tactics for Boredom

1. Call or text someone on your team and figure out something fun or relaxing to do.
2. Give yourself a project or hobby: Play a video game, build something, start a collection, clean out the closet, whatever you need to do to keep your mind busy.

3. Chew gum and drink water.

4. Volunteer for a service event in your area.

Tactics for Holidays and Events

1. For anniversaries and birthdays, eat ahead of time and come with a full stomach. Just like social gatherings, keep a glass of water, soda water, or diet soda in hand. Chew gum. Avoid the food as much as possible.

2. Also see tactics for social gatherings and people triggers.

Call to Action

On the left side, write your top 3 event triggers, and on the right side, write the tactics you will use to navigate around it or through it!

Top 3 event triggers	Top 5 tactics you can use
1.	1. 2. 3. 4. 5.
2.	1. 2. 3. 4. 5.
3.	1. 2. 3. 4. 5.

Why Am I Always Hungry?

Do you ever consume thousands of calories in a sitting, and then feel hungry again within just minutes or hours? It can be so frustrating and depressing feeling like your body is an out-of-control eating machine. Many people have lost touch with their true hunger and become slaves to their emotional hunger.

There is a huge difference between the feeling of physical fullness and feeling emotionally satisfied. However, the wiring in our brains often gets crossed so that it is difficult to distinguish between the two. Through years of poor eating habits in response to emotional triggers, yo-yo dieting, and bouts of binge eating we can confuse the brain to think that loneliness and depression are hunger, and the act of eating is comfort.

This can lead to the endless consumption of thousands of calories. While your body may be full and satisfied, your emotions are not...so you continue to mindlessly eat, searching for a comfort of fullness that may never come... until you are ready to stop, take a moment, and pay attention to what is *really* going on.

It is easy to get stuck on autopilot and find yourself "blind bingeing" on junk foods. However, you need to:

- Relearn what true hunger feels like.
- Before you eat anything, stop and ask yourself, *"Am I really hungry?"*
- Log your foods.

Reality Check

Your triggers aren't going anywhere. They are a part of life, and will be present to test you every day. However, the more aware and prepared you are, the greater the chance you will overcome them.

DAY 21

It's Time to Weigh In

Your End-of-Cycle Weight: _____

At this time, feel free to take any other measurements as well and note them here: _____.

Day 21: Reset Day

It's Reset Day! Make meals easy by cooking up our Clean Cheat recipes (see suggested menu below), or simply add 1,000 extra calories of foods you love to a normal high-carb day.

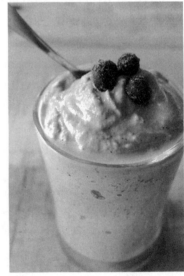

Meal 1: Candied Pecan Protein Waffles

Meal 2: Sweet Potato Nachos

Meal 3: Banana Berry Ice Cream

Meal 4: Pigs in a Blanket

Meal 5: One-Minute Brownie

Rest Day

Now relax! Take the day off and rest—no Metabolic Missions and no Accelerators!

LESSON 21
LIVE WITH PURPOSE

Man is a goal seeking animal. His life only has meaning if he is reaching out and striving for his goals.

—Aristotle

Right now, you may be solely driven by your own personal goals, wants, and needs—which is totally awesome. Remember, in order to change you must be beneficially selfish! Setting *your* goals and declaring *your* dream has given you a direction and a purpose. And now, 21 days or more into your journey, you are seeing and feeling the difference in your life. However, to make this "difference" lifelong, we want to ask you to open up your mind to something that may seem a bit counterintuitive...

We want to ask you to begin to open your mind to the value that you can bring to others' lives. In his *7 Habits of Highly Effective People*, the great Stephen Covey wrote about the distinctions among dependence, independence, and interdependence.

We are programmed to be interdependent with others—to contribute to our family, community, and society—and when we make this connection real, we not only help others but also maximize our sense of value and belonging. When we have a contributing purpose in life, it satisfies and fulfills us on a whole new level.

In many ways, this process of transformation is akin to the process of rehabilitation, and one of the most powerful steps in true recovery is when a person becomes a sponsor to help others through their journeys. That's what we have in mind here.

So what if you could make a positive impact in someone else's life? Or many people's lives? You can. Transformation is not just about changing your life, but also about being the catalyst for change in others. In the most beneficially selfish way, reaching out to others—to help, guide, or inspire—helps keep you living a life of transformation without sliding back into your old destructive habits, and so keeps you from gaining the weight back.

Call to Action:
Become a Weight Loss Superstar

Start thinking about the impact that you are going to make in the world. Whether you have reached your goal in just one 21-day phase or several phases, there are millions of people out there who want to do what you have just done. You can be their motivation! Want to know where everyone is? Online. Hundreds of millions of people want to hear from you! Here are some other ideas for reaching out to others:

- Build a social media following: Start an Instagram, Facebook, and Twitter account. Follow and "like" other weight loss accounts and amazing success stories.
- Post your before and weekly pics to chart your progress for everyone.
- Post motivational quotes that resonate with you throughout your journey.
- Share the lessons of transformation that resonate most with you. Be real and vulnerable—talk about struggles you encountered during the process and struggles you currently deal with today.
- Post recipes and exercises that you love.
- Post tips and tricks that work for you on the journey.

This isn't a ploy to get free social media. In fact, we don't care for any credit. All we want for you is to live a healthier and happier life. If you have changed your life, or are in the process of change, all we ask is that you help others through the journey. Whether it is your closest friends and family, or your online community, teaching and guiding others will engrain the lessons of transformation into your life.

This is why we have dedicated our lives to helping others. It enriches our lives beyond measure. But don't take our word for it—you just have to experience it for yourself!

POWELL

PHASE ONE'S DONE: NOW WHAT?

Congratulations on completing a 21-day phase of Extreme Transformation!

If you have reached your weight loss goal, we are so darn proud of you! Very well done! ☺

If you are still on your weight loss journey, then let's get fired up to do this again!

If you are losing weight consistently and comfortably on the Extreme Cycle, then keep everything going exactly as you have been doing it. As they say, "If it ain't broke, don't fix it!"

However, if your weight loss begins to slow at any time, there are two powerful cycles that we use to jump-start your weight loss again:

Turbocharge the Extreme Cycle

If after a full 21 days of the Extreme Cycle you aren't dropping as fast as you should or want to, we turbocharge the cycle. Replace two of the high-carb days with low-carb days. We call this the "Turbo Cycle." This is what it looks like:

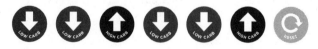

After your first 21-day phase, feel free to drop into the Turbo Cycle if you really want to speed things up.

The Slingshot

If you have completed several 21-day Extreme Cycle phases, have already dropped down to the Turbo Cycle, and your weight loss has still significantly slowed or stopped, it is time for the ultimate Reset. This approach we call the Slingshot seems totally unorthodox but works like a charm to trick your body into losing weight again. Your body has likely adapted to the calorie deficit and increased activity. We have written extensively about this process in our previous books, *Choose to Lose* and *Choose More, Lose More for Life*.

Essentially, the Slingshot is a week of consecutive high-carb days—each day with double the carbs! A week doing the Slingshot looks like this:

Day 1: High-Carb Day (double your carb portion every meal)

Day 2: High-Carb Day (double your carb portion every meal)

Day 3: High-Carb Day (double your carb portion every meal)

Day 4: High-Carb Day (double your carb portion every meal)

Day 5: High-Carb Day (double your carb portion every meal)

Day 6: High-Carb Day (double your carb portion every meal)

Day 7: High-Carb Day (double your carb portion every meal)

After the Slingshot, drop back into the Extreme Cycle or Turbo Cycle and watch your weight drop like a rock again!

PART 3

Your New Life

EMBRACING THE NEW YOU: MASTERING MAINTENANCE

A *huge* congratulations! Completing your Extreme Transformation is an incredible feat. It is physically, mentally, and emotionally challenging—yet unbelievably empowering in every aspect of your life. Along the way, you've lost the weight, you've come to feel more energetic, and most importantly you have created love and belief in yourself! You now know that you can do anything you set your mind to...and that you've been worth it all along. We are so proud of you.

You've been working the lessons like a warrior and we know that you feel accomplished and alive. But just like all things in life that are of value, this incredible sense of self-esteem, confidence, and love will not last forever—unless you work at it. That's what real maintenance is all about.

First, let's define what maintenance means: It's "an active process of ensuring that the necessities for a new or current state continue." Just as it takes nourishment and maintenance to keep your lawn green and your flowers in bloom, it also takes nourishment and maintenance to keep this new state of awesomeness you are now living. You must actively eat and exercise to stay at the weight you have achieved. You must also practice the lessons of transformation daily. Maintenance doesn't have to be a time-consuming process—it takes just minutes a day—but the fact remains that you still need to be beneficially selfish and spend some time and energy on yourself and your well-being every day.

In this chapter, we will lay out for you the pitfalls ahead, tell you what to expect, and help you create a bulletproof strategy to keep the weight off for years to come.

Reality Check

If you now feel like you've completed your Extreme Transformation and believe that the process is over so you can "go back to normal"—you are very wrong. Let's not forget where living a so-called "normal" life got you last time. The majority of people who allow that mind-set to persist will spiral right back to where they started.

Remember: Transformation is a new lifestyle, not a diet that begins and ends. In other words, there is no end to your new life—it will continue forever, if you let it. Our goal is to help you find a new normal within these pages—a way to remain committed to bettering yourself and constantly striving for optimal health and happiness.

So here we are at a proverbial fork in the road. If you go in one direction, it will lead you right back to where you were. The frustration, the depression, the weight.

If you go in the other direction, it will lead you to a life of new food and physical experiences, new opportunities, and new possibilities at your ideal weight. Ten, twenty, thirty years from now, you'll still be living life at a lean and healthy weight. It is totally possible.

If you choose to continue in the direction that will lead to a fit and healthy life, we say this: Welcome to your new normal! Let's explore this new journey—to sustain your weight loss, live a happy, balanced life, and integrate some of our best tricks of the trade to handle the inevitable obstacles and challenges that lie ahead.

Read closely. This is how we do it.

ACTIONS FOR MAINTENANCE

These **8 Actions** will help you maintain your weight loss and feel great!

Declare Your New Goal

All of us need direction. We constantly need something to work toward. Without a goal, a purpose, it's easy to slip into a state of despair. And in despair we quickly find ourselves grasping for the comforts we once relied on to feel good and back in the grips of our vice—food.

To avoid this situation, immediately upon reaching your weight loss goal you need to have the next goal in place. Our brain needs something to strive for and a new goal or purpose to keep us happy. Think of it like that scene in *Raiders of the Lost Ark*, when Indiana Jones has to quickly switch out the gold statue with a sandbag—we've got to quickly trade your addiction again into something your brain likes for maintenance.

Over your weight loss journey, you have felt the thrill of seeing the numbers drop on the scale and squeezing into new clothes. You received accolades from your family, friends, and co-workers on a regular basis. These are payoffs you experience on a regular basis—and your brain processes these payoffs as rewards. As Bruce recalls, "Losing weight was awesome because it was always high fives and hugs from everyone. Now, nobody ever comes up to me and says, 'Bro! You're killing it in maintenance!' Or, 'Great job. You look the same!'" Now it's time to maintain because the compliments will most likely dwindle or even stop. Your clothing size will probably regulate. And the number on the scale will more or less remain the same. The satisfaction that you gained from these changes will begin to peter out and the reality of maintenance will set in.

For many, the thought of regular daily workouts for the rest of their lives can feel daunting—like an endless cycle. Let's be honest, working out just to work out can often seem more like torture. But *training* for something is totally different! We train for a payoff. Everyone we coach through maintenance continues to train for *something* to keep it fun and exciting—they regularly sign up for community events like 5Ks, triathlons, marathons, mud runs—any kind of activity to keep them getting fitter, feeling better, and thriving in their fitness community... but most important to keep them training toward another goal.

So what do you want to do?

Increase your strength? Get six-pack abs? Run a marathon? Enter a body-building contest or a CrossFit competition? Rock a slammin' body for spring break or your upcoming vacay? Your goals are limitless, and the best part is that once you reach one goal, you will always have another within reach! Whatever you choose, declare a new goal *now*, and make it SMART!

What are you going to accomplish next?

What does it look like? (Describe what it will take to achieve this goal and how you will feel when you reach it.)

When are you going to accomplish it?

Once again, surround yourself with reminders of what you will achieve next and let everyone know your new commitment. Place pictures, clothes, whatever around your house, car, workplace...everywhere!

If it's an event, sign up weeks or months in advance. Heck, sign up for several!

Chris Tip

Aside from physical fitness goals, there are other incredibly powerful motivators to help engrain the maintenance lifestyle:

- Date other fitness-minded people.
- Start a weight loss website or blog.
- Begin a new career that supports your new lifestyle.
- Get involved with your community, charity, or church.

As dedicated foodies, Hannah and her husband had to replace almost all of their social activities involving food. Instead of chasing the best new restaurant, they joined a basketball league and play sand volleyball Wednesday nights. They also joined an online culinary course to learn healthy new recipes that fit into their new lifestyle!

The more you can submerge yourself in the fitness community, the greater your chances for lifelong success...oh, and you'll also meet the nicest, friendliest, most caring people in the world!

Review Your Support System

You've had at least 21 days to help identify who's really on your team, including your superfriend. Maybe some of your teammates have come and some have gone in that time. Whoever is on your team now will be needed just as much or more during maintenance! Sit down and communicate openly with them about your new goals and aspirations. Get them involved. They can even commit to your new maintenance activities and goals with you!

Keep Doing the Extreme Cycle

Here's the deal. Your body still needs real, whole natural food. You still need to eat five times a day and drink plenty of water. This is for your overall health and well-being! Guys, you will need approximately 2,000 to 2,500 calories to maintain. This number can increase to 2,500 to 3,000 after about six months as your body stabilizes.

Ladies, you need approximately 1,500 calories to maintain. This number can go up to between 1,700 to 2,000 calories after six months as your body stabilizes.

The number of calories goes up or down according to how much you exercise on a daily and weekly basis, and your new physique or fitness goals.

Following the Extreme Cycle during maintenance will keep you eating five meals every day, each made up of good-quality food, and drinking plenty of water. However, there is more flexibility for introducing new foods into your lifestyle. During maintenance (and weight loss) we strongly recommend downloading a calorie tracker on your phone to monitor your daily food intake. New trackers are insanely easy to use and take literally seconds to log your food. This is what we have *all* of our participants do, and they swear by it!

And don't worry: Reset days and meals will still exist. Your body and mind will get the foods they need and crave to avoid that feeling of deprivation, even during maintenance.

Select Your Reset Meals with Lifestyle Layers

The reset meal structure of the 21-Day Extreme Cycle may have worked perfectly for you. If rewarding yourself once a week after six days of clean eating felt good emotionally, physically, and mentally, then do not change how you reward yourself. However, if you felt deprived or restricted at all during the actual weight loss portion of the Extreme Cycle, and you feel hesitant about your ability to succeed and continue with this structure in maintenance, then it may be time to change things up a little for this next phase. Do not worry.

In this new phase of life, it is acceptable to customize your reward days, following the guidelines below, so that you feel completely physically satiated, fulfilled, and satisfied. Otherwise, maintenance will be difficult to sustain.

We call these regular rewards that are laced throughout our days "Lifestyle Layers." The layering concept relates to the idea that you will simply "lay down" more and more rewards throughout your day and week until you feel totally satisfied throughout your days, giving you the confidence to make it a long-term lifestyle.

Choose Your Layers

Decide how many layers work for you. Here are your options:

- **Once a Week**—If you felt totally satisfied while Extreme Cycling and can maintain that pattern indefinitely, then feel free to indulge in a big reward day once a week…for life!
- **Twice a Week**—Pick two days to reward yourself. Try splitting them up, like Wednesday and Sunday.
- **Every Other Day**—If you can't have it today, you can always have it tomorrow!
- **One to Three "Daily Hugs" a Day**—First thing in the morning or later in the day, a small daily reward or two always gives us something to look forward to. Think a sugar-free candy, or low-cal specialty coffee.

Whatever you do, *do not* select to reward yourself *less* than what will satisfy you. This will lead to feelings of deprivation and inevitably going back to old destructive eating patterns. The *right* way to do maintenance is to keep laying down Lifestyle Layers until you feel satisfied, but keeping it within your calorie range!

Heidi Tip

If at any time during maintenance you find the number on the scale creeping back up, simply remove one or two of your Lifestyle Layers and Extreme Cycle yourself right back down. You did it once, you can do it again!

Plan Your Rewards

When it's time to indulge during maintenance, don't blindly wander through the days succumbing to drive-thrus and donuts that Bob from accounting brought into the office. You'll quickly find yourself pushing the parameters of maintenance.

When you plan your Lifestyle Layers, put some thought into it and treat yourself to some quality eats—because you deserve it. Maybe it's some dark chocolate, or a caramel latte from a fancy coffee shop. Think about your five favorite reward foods and list them with the portion you feel comfortable eating. Next, using the new calorie tracking app that we requested you to download, write the calorie impact of that food on the right hand side.

Favorite Reward Food	Portion Size	Calories

Not that you have to eat from this list all of the time, but whatever you choose to indulge in, know the calorie impact and how it fits into your daily maintenance range.

Keep Moving

For exercise, you should continue to do at least 30 minutes of moderate to intense activity daily. However, if 30 minutes is not attainable every day, then reduce your commitment to something you *know* you can do.

Maybe just start by Accelerating for 5 to 15 minutes a day again. Maybe just do one Metabolic Mission a day instead of Accelerators. As long as you keep your promises and keep moving, you will win in the long run!

Weigh In Daily

During maintenance, weigh-ins change. It is extremely important that you weigh in at the beginning of *every* day. Start your day creating an awareness for the maintenance task at hand. While this advice may be controversial for some who worry about fixating on the scale, research has recently found that those who weigh in daily keep the weight off longer—or for life. You choose!

The Winning Range

Research has shown that individuals who can keep their weight within a 10-pound range for over five years have a 90 percent chance of lifelong success! Give yourself an acceptable range to stay within—plus or minus 5 pounds.

My upper weight range limit for maintenance is: _____

My lower weight range limit for maintenance is: _____

Put your upper and lower range on paper and post it somewhere you will see it every day!

Keep Taking Pictures!

Take pics of yourself weekly. Many people who have lost a significant amount of weight report still "seeing" their larger selves when they look in the mirror. Research has proven that it can take up to five years for your brain to "catch up" to the realization of your new weight. To keep a realistic view of your new body and stay motivated, take weekly pics and compare them!

INTEGRITY IS ALWAYS THE SECRET

Building your integrity is the true secret path to dignity and ultimately losing the weight—and it is the *exact* same for maintenance. In this new chapter of your life, we set new goals, make new commitments and promises, and keep them every day. Just as keeping these promises will propel you to an extraordinary way of life and well-being, breaking these promises will do the exact opposite—they will completely derail you. Whether losing weight or keeping it off forever, your ultimate well-being will always boil down to this:

Integrity: Do what you say you're going to do, when you say you're going to do it.

One Broken Promise Can Lead to Backslide

A lot of people lose weight. Many of them gain it back. We've all seen it—maybe it was a friend, a family member, a co-worker, or possibly even you.

We are going to teach you something very important here: Every single weight regain can be traced back to a single broken promise—a time when you didn't do what you said you were going to do, which was then followed by an internal dialogue of excuses and lies to continue to rationalize the destructive behavior. The following is a typical story of weight regain. We have dissected it so that you can see the moment integrity was broken, and how quickly the internal dialogue enabled a destructive behavior. Pay close attention; it may seem eerily familiar!

Shari's Story

Shari lost 62 pounds over six months following the Extreme Cycle and Metabolic Missions.

Her promise: "In maintenance, I will continue to follow the Extreme Cycle and Metabolic Missions with my new added daily Lifestyle Layers to keep me satisfied and fulfilled."

Her reality: "A few weeks after hitting my goal, I felt good and on top of the world. I felt like I had weight loss and maintenance all figured out and nothing could take me down. One night, I was at a work cocktail party and kept making trips back to the bar and buffet, even though it was *way* off my maintenance plan and far beyond my Lifestyle Layers."

Her internal excuse: "I am in better shape than most of these people. I deserve to indulge here and there."

Her downslide: "A couple of days later, I was starving and stopped at a fast-food drive-thru for lunch."

Her internal excuse: "I've got this. C'mon, I've lost 62 pounds. I know what I'm doing. Plus, I worked out today."

Her further downslide: "Fast food once a day became a daily routine for me beyond my Daily Hugs and then led to more splurges in the evening. My clothes started to get tight and I was too terrified to step on the scale."

Her internal lie: "It isn't about the number on the scale anymore for me, it's about how I look and feel."

A further downslide: "Just a couple of months later I mustered up the courage to step on the scale after my clothes weren't fitting anymore, and I had gained 43 pounds back."

Reading the story, you can see numerous lessons of transformation popping out: Shari lost sight of the hidden path, she's not keeping her promises, she's not being vulnerable and authentic, she's not falling without failing to stop the downslide...the list goes on!

Whether it's eating a whole bucket of popcorn at the movies or finishing half of a pizza at your kid's party—the rules of maintenance are the same as the rules of weight loss: To get back on track and prevent sliding further downward, you must confess, reassess, and recommit. You *must* be aware of the dangerous internal conversations that follow the broken promise, full of excuses and lies. Because it always leads back to the bingeing, back to the loss of control, and back to the old you.

Nobody wants to be that cautionary tale of weight regain. We hope we've got your attention because this is the unfortunate and all-too-common reality of life after weight loss. The good news is that with your awareness, it doesn't have to happen!

BEWARE YOUR INNER VOICE

Sometimes the first slip-up (broken promise) in maintenance is a mistake and not intentional. Sometimes it happens and we don't even realize it until later. Sometimes it seems so minuscule that you'd only be wasting someone's time to tell them about it. Doesn't matter. Once you identify the broken promise, it has to be healed. Heck, a quick phone call or three-line text to a superfriend can upright the ship in a heartbeat.

> *Messed up. Ate way too much and feel horrible about it. Recommitting now and will keep my promise to eat on plan.*

However, if the confession doesn't happen and you begin to find yourself slipping more and more…let "internal dialogue warnings" help identify when you are in a downslide situation. Here are some more dangerous internal excuses and lies that you should be aware of, and their inevitable reality. They can, and probably will, come up any day in maintenance:

Internal Dialogue: "It's finally over and I can go back to 'normal.'"

Reality: Don't forget where your old normal got you in the first place. You'll gain most, if not all, of the weight back. This way of living should be your new normal!

Internal Dialogue: "I'm going to do a muscle-bulking phase."

Reality: Addicts usually can't bulk under control. You'll be up 50 pounds before you know it. (See Lesson 20, Triggers and Tactics.)

Internal Dialogue: "I'll adjust my maintenance window 10 pounds higher because I like the way I am now."

Reality: You're only saying this because you've gained weight and don't want to put in the work to get back to your true 10-pound window. You're in a dangerous mind-set here. You're protecting your addiction, and will raise the window again as you keep gaining weight back.

Internal Dialogue: "It'll be nice to have some curves back."

Reality: Those aren't curves, it's body fat. If you want curves, lift some weight and make them *real* curves.

Internal Dialogue: "I messed up, but I'm an inspiration. I can't let them down by admitting my mistakes. They'll think less of me."

Reality: Don't get so stuck in an identity that prevents you from being great—true heroes confess, reassess, and recommit. (See Lesson 9, Be Open, Honest, and Vulnerable.) Trust us. You might be surprised at the support others give when you are authentic and share your mistakes—even coming from someone whom they consider an inspiration.

Internal Dialogue: "I saw Becky eating that junk food and she looks amazing! If she can eat that way, then I can, too, and get away with it."

Reality: You don't know *exactly* how much Becky eats or exercises during the day, so you cannot assume she's "getting away" with anything. Plus, if Becky is early in maintenance, she may be starting a slippery downward spiral. Addicts feed off other addicts to rationalize and fuel destructive behavior. Be careful.

Internal Dialogue: "I can eat this because at least I'm still smaller than Terry."

Reality: You are comparing yourself to others' weaknesses to rationalize and protect your own destructive behavior. That's not okay. You are better than that and you know it. (See Lesson 8: Believe in Yourself.)

Internal Dialogue: "I worked out extra hard today, so I've earned additional calories."

Reality: If it isn't one of your Daily Hugs, you haven't earned it. Be careful. Justification after a hard workout is a trap we can get caught in all too often. See Lesson 20: Triggers and Tactics.

What's our point here? Your inner dialogue will be around forever. Stay in touch with it and be on the lookout for negative self-talk, excuses, and other ways to rationalize breaking promises to yourself. If you're human like us, temptation will spark the voice every day. The moral of the story is that your promises *always* come first. If you end up breaking a promise, the downward spiral begins. Remember: The downward spiral doesn't have to continue. Simply confess, reassess, recommit, and get back on track to the rest of your life.

MASTERING MAINTENANCE

As you embark upon a whole new journey of maintenance, take to heart the powerful and universal lessons you learned during your weight loss journey. We strongly advise you to *re*-learn, *re*-love, and *re*-live the 21 powerful lessons you learned during your weight loss, because they apply to your maintenance success as well! We reflect on at least one lesson every day. As Dr. Holly likes to remind our *Extreme Weight Loss* peeps, "Maintenance is a process even greater than weight loss." As her research indicates, people who not only lose weight but keep it off are those who "master" the lessons in maintenance.

Keep in mind that nobody does maintenance perfectly. However, as long as you stay connected with your support team, declare your goals, keep your promises, and stay true and vulnerable with yourself and your lifelong transformation journey, then you will always succeed. The journey of maintenance is nearly identical to the journey of weight loss. The only difference is a new goal and a few more calories. That's it.

A heartfelt welcome to the rest of your life. ☺

Chris & Heidi

PART 4

The Metabolic Movements

What follows is a detailed guide to all the Metabolic Movements used in the daily Missions.

METABOLIC MISSION WARM-UP

Before your Metabolic Mission, perform this brief warm-up.

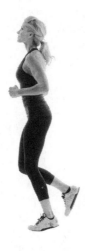

30 seconds jogging in place

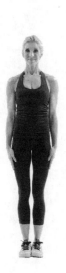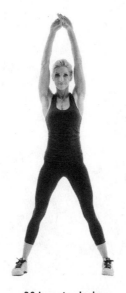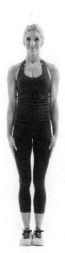

30 Jumping Jacks

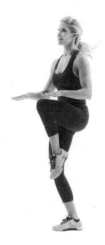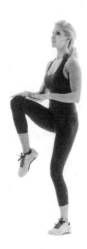

30 seconds High Knees

Then perform 10 repetitions each of the following movements. Hold each position for a brief 1–2 seconds to feel the stretch, then continue.

Twisters

Perform 10 reps of this movement.

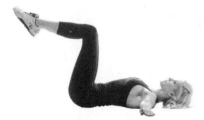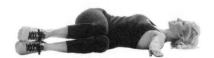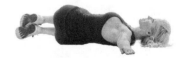

Begin lying on the floor faceup, knees and hips at a 90-degree angle as if you are sitting in a chair, arms extended to your sides.

Keeping your shoulders anchored to the floor and knees together, rotate your legs over to the left side. Touch your left knee to the floor to make a complete repetition.

Rotate your legs over to the right side and touch your right knee to the floor to make another repetition.

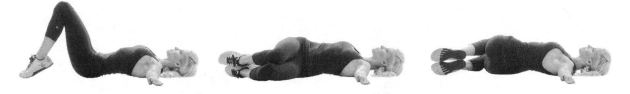

Modification: Keep your toes on the floor while rotating the knees back and forth.

Swoops

Perform 10 reps of this movement.

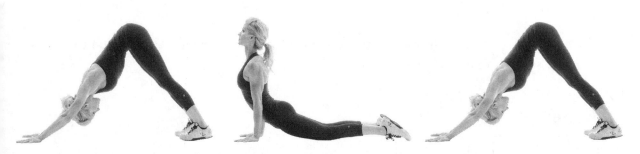

Begin in the high pike position, tucking your head between your shoulders and driving your heels into the floor.

Shift your body forward, lowering your hips to the floor. Press your shoulders down and away from your ears as you stretch your abs.

Press back into the high pike position.

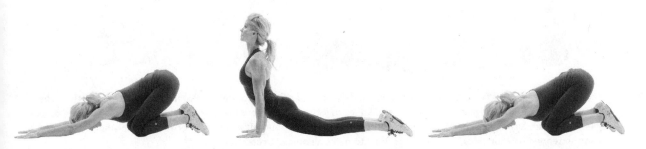

Modification: Instead of performing the movement on your feet, do it from your knees.

Lunge Stretches

Perform 10 reps of this alternating movement.

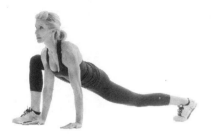
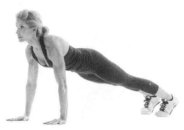
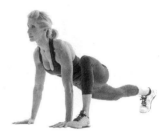

Place one foot behind you in a deep runner's lunge, keeping the back knee off the floor. Place hands on the floor inside the front knee. Shift your weight onto your front heel and feel a deep stretch in the opposition hip flexor.

Switch legs, keeping knees off the floor.

Repeat on the other side.

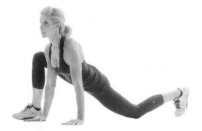
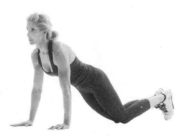
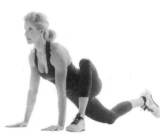

Modification: Start from your knees and alternate by placing your knees on the floor to transition into the stretch.

Here are detailed instructions for each Metabolic Movement.

AIR SQUATS

Rules for the rep to count: At the bottom of the Air Squat, the crease of your hip must pass below the top of the kneecap. At the top of the movement, the hips and knees must be fully extended, standing upright.

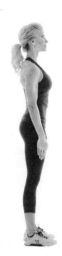
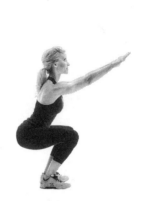
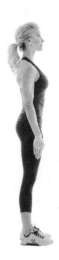

Begin in a standing position, feet shoulder width apart, toes pointed slightly out from parallel.

Keeping your weight in your heels, bend your knees and lower your buttocks down and back, as if you're being pulled backward from a belt. Reach your arms upward as the crease of your hips drops, making sure that your knees are tracking directly over your toes (not inward).

Drive upward through your heels, standing back up to the beginning position with your knees and hips extended.

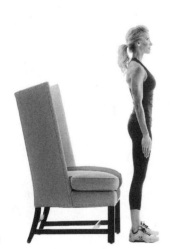
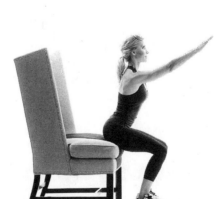
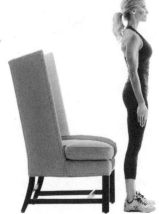

Modification: To make the exercise easier, use a chair to support the bottom of your squat. Buttocks must touch the chair.

BACK LUNGES

Rules for the rep to count: At the bottom of the lunge, your back knee must gently "kiss" the floor. At the top of the movement, you must be standing upright with your hips and knees extended.

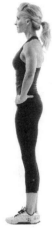
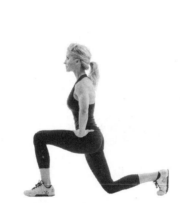
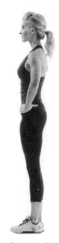

Begin in a standing position.

Take an aggressive step backward with your right foot, gently "kissing" your back knee to the floor.

Keeping your front left knee over the toe, drive the forward heel to a standing position.

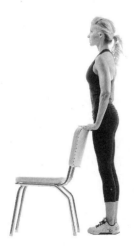
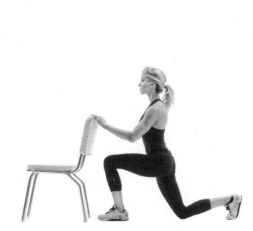
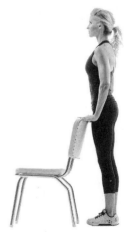

Modification: To make the exercise easier, grab onto a chair or other object for stability. When lunging, let the back knee go as low as possible, but stay in a pain-free range of motion.

BURPEES (series)

Rules for the rep to count: You may get down to the floor however you choose, but your chest and thighs must touch the floor at the bottom of the movement, and your feet must leave the floor and hands touch overhead at the top.

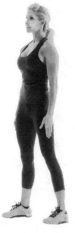

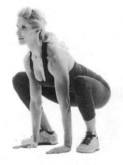

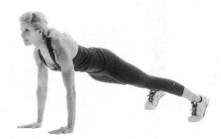

Begin standing with your feet at shoulder width.

Squat down and place your hands on the floor just inside your feet.

Jump back to a plank position.

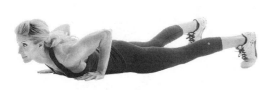

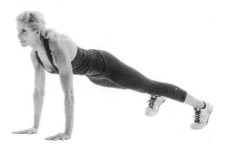

Perform a Push-Up.

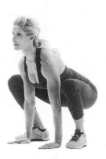

Jump forward with your feet
outside your hands.

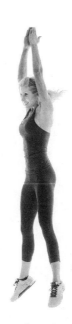

Jump up and touch your
hands overhead.

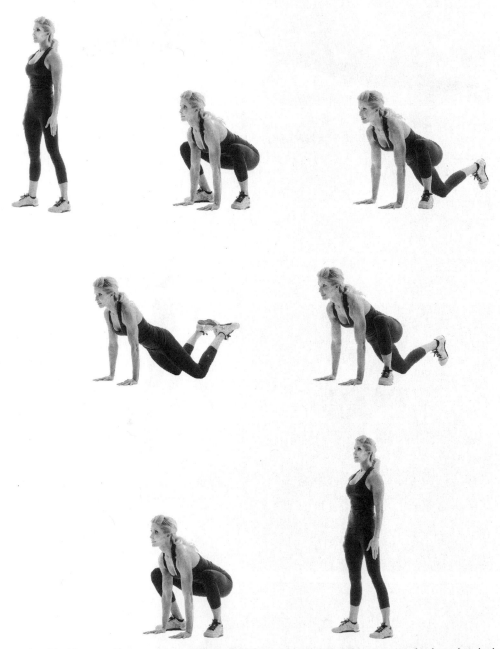

Modification: If you need to make the Burpees easier, drop to a knee or step back to the plank position. The Push-Up portion can be done from the knees or by keeping the hips on the floor. Simply stand up at the end to complete the Burpee.

FLUTTERKICKS

Rules for the rep to count: Your knees must be extended with both feet off the floor. The heel of your top foot must rise above the toe of your bottom foot. Both legs must kick for the rep to count.

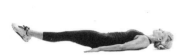 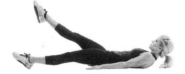 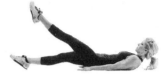

Begin lying on your back with your hands wedged under your hips. Keeping your knees extended, tighten your core and raise your feet 1 to 2 feet off the floor.

Alternate raising and lowering your legs in a "scissor kick" rhythmic motion.

Modification: Allow one heel to touch the floor while raising the other leg.

HIGH KNEES

Rules for the rep to count: Elbows must remain at a 90-degree angle. The top of your knee must touch your hand for the rep to count.

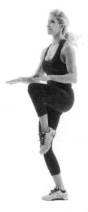 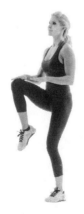 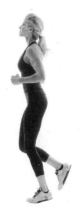

Keeping your weight on your toes, stand tall with your abs engaged. Alternate driving your knees upward toward your chest at a running tempo.

Keeping your elbows bent at 90 degrees, drive with your knees until they touch your hands.

Modification: Jog in place.

HOLLOW ROCKS

Rules for the rep to count: At the bottom of the movement, your arms must be straight overhead and your heels must be raised at least a foot above the floor. At the top of the movement, arms must be straight overhead and your torso must be raised at least a foot off the floor.

Begin lying on your back with your arms overhead.

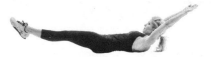

Lying on your back, tighten your abs and raise your arms and legs 1 to 2 feet off the floor, creating a "hollow body" position.

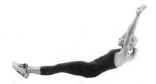

Keeping your core tight and your body rigid, allow your heels to lower back down to the floor, raising your torso off the floor.

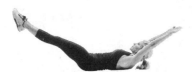

Rock back and forth in a rhythmic motion. Modification for upper body only.

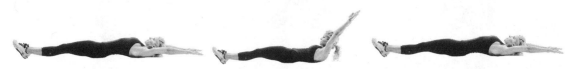

Modification: Leave your heels on the floor and perform the movement using just your upper body.

JUMPING JACKS

Rules for the rep to count: At the top of the movement you must be standing upright and hands must be touching the sides of your thighs. At the bottom of the movement, hands must touch overhead while feet land in a position wider than your shoulders.

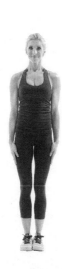 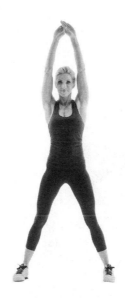 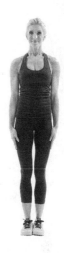

Begin in a standing position, feet together and hands at your sides.	In one motion, jump feet out to a wide stance and clap hands overhead.	Jump feet back together, bringing arms quickly back down to your sides.

Modification: Instead of jumping, step a leg out to the side.

KICKBACKS

Rules for rep to count: At the bottom of the Kickback, your hips must be fully extended with just your hands and feet touching the floor. At the top of the movement, your hips and knees must be fully extended standing upright.

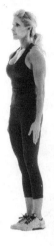

Begin standing with your feet together or at shoulder width.

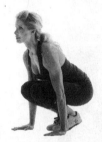

Squat down and place your hands on the floor just outside your feet.

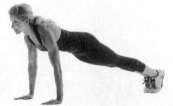

Step or jump your feet back to a Push-Up position.

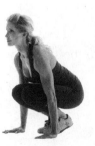

Jump forward with your feet landing outside your hands.

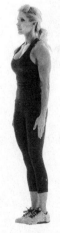

Stand straight up.

Modification: To make the exercise easier, step your feet back to the plank position instead of jumping.

LEG LEVERS

Rules for the rep to count: At the bottom of the Leg Lever, the heels must touch the floor with the knees extended. At the top of the movement, with knees extended, the feet must pass through a vertical plane directly over your head.

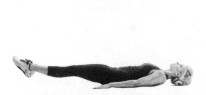 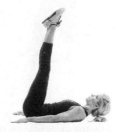 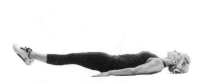

Begin lying on your back with your arms braced against the floor (or holding a chair or sofa), heels touching the floor.

Keeping your knees extended, raise your legs upward until your feet are directly overhead.

Lower your heels to the floor.

Modification: Simply alternate legs, keeping one leg on the floor and raising the other, then switch. Each leg (right and left) must raise once to count as a single rep.

MOUNTAIN CLIMBERS (series)

Rules for rep to count: The forward foot must touch the floor at a point above the mid-shin of the back leg.

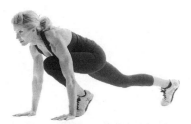

Begin in a deep runner's stance with both hands on the floor, shoulder width apart.

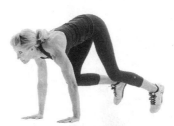

Keeping your abs tight, jump and switch as fast as you can.

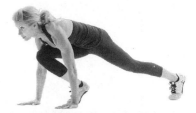

Land gently with the opposite foot forward. As soon as your feet touch down, jump quickly and switch feet again. Switch your feet back and forth in a rhythmic motion.

Modification: To make the exercise easier, don't jump between Mountain Climbers. Just step and touch—then switch.

PUSH-UPS

Rules for the rep to count: At the bottom of the Push-Up, your chest and thighs must touch the floor. At the top of the Push-Up, your elbows must be fully extended.

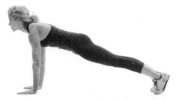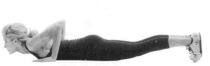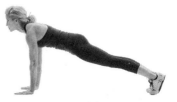

Begin in the plank position, hands underneath your shoulders, elbows extended and abs tight.

Bend at your elbows, lowering your body to the floor but staying rigid from your feet to your shoulders.

Immediately press upward extending your elbows, keeping your abs tight and your body rigid from your toes.

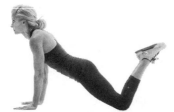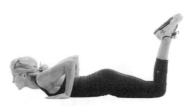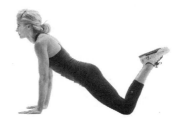

Modification 1: If you need an intermediate level Push-Up, try them from your knees.

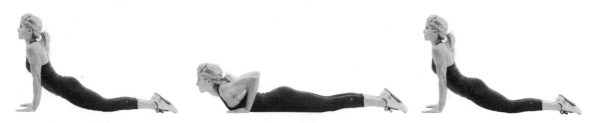

Modification 2: If you need a beginner level Push-Up, leave your hips on the floor and allow your back to extend as you press off of the floor.

SIT-UPS

Rules for the rep to count: With legs either straight or bent, hands must touch the floor above your head at the bottom of the movement, then touch your feet at the top of the movement.

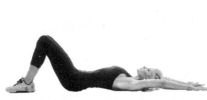 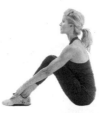 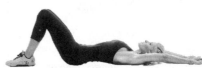

Begin by lying on the floor faceup, knees bent, feet flat on the floor, and arms extended overhead.

Swing your arms forward, using the momentum to raise your shoulders and torso off the floor. Touch your toes.

Extend your arms overhead as you lower your torso and shoulders back to the floor. Touch the floor overhead to complete the repetition.

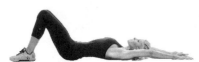 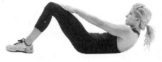 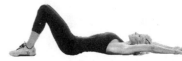

Modification 1: For a beginner Sit-Up, touch your fingers to your knees to mark the top of the rep.

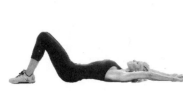 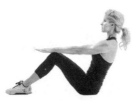 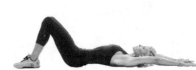

Modification 2: For an intermediate Sit-Up, touch your wrists to your knees to mark the top of the rep.

PART 5

Extreme Cycle Recipes

Although some of these recipes may seem fancy and gourmet, you don't need to be an Iron Chef to make them! If you're new to preparing your own food, don't worry—we've made it insanely simple for you. For each and every week of this program, we have created:

- A shopping list, for quick and easy grocery shopping for that week's worth of recipes.
- A meal prep guide for every three days of the program, to keep preparation for each meal to just a few minutes.
- A bulk prep cooking guide, for multiple cooking options for all of your foods.

These guides will teach you the necessary skills to conveniently prepare delicious food for the rest of your life! You'll find these step-by-step guides in the Appendices.

Note: For all recipes, 1 serving is the yield unless otherwise specified.

BREAKFASTS

Apple Cinnamon Muesli

Breakfast

⅓ cup rolled oats (½ cup for men)

½ cup unsweetened almond milk (¾ cup for men)

1 tablespoon fat-free plain Greek yogurt (2 tablespoons for men)

¼ cup vanilla protein powder (½ cup for men)

Dash of cinnamon

½ apple, chopped

1 tablespoon sliced almonds

Vanilla stevia drops to taste

Mix oats, almond milk, yogurt, protein powder, and cinnamon together in a bowl or in a mason jar. Top with chopped apples and sliced almonds.

Store in the fridge overnight. Eat cold. Add stevia for desired sweetness.

Women: 280 cals; 8g fat; 35g carb; 20g protein
Men: 420 cals; 11g fat; 47g carb; 37g protein

Banana Yogurt Parfait and Pumpkin Seed Granola

Breakfast

Parfait

1 cup fat-free plain Greek yogurt

1 ripe banana, sliced

1 tablespoon Pumpkin Seed Granola (3 tablespoons for men)

Truvia (optional)

Top Greek yogurt and with sliced banana and Pumpkin Seed Granola (recipe follows). Option: add some Truvia to cut the sourness of the yogurt.

Pumpkin Seed Granola

1 teaspoon extra-virgin coconut oil

¼ cup slivered almonds, raw and unsalted

¼ cup raw, unsalted pumpkin seeds

½ teaspoon Truvia sweetener

¼ teaspoon ground cinnamon or pumpkin pie spice

Pinch of ground nutmeg

Pinch of salt substitute

Heat the coconut oil in nonstick skillet over medium heat.

Toss the almonds and pumpkin seeds in coconut oil and stir to avoid burning.

Add Truvia, cinnamon, nutmeg, and salt substitute, and mix.

Makes 1 serving, with leftover granola

Women: 290 cals; 4g fat; 39g carb; 27g protein

Men: 385 cals; 12g fat; 42g carb; 30g protein

Breakfast Frittata Veggie "Muffins"

Breakfast

2 tablespoons extra-virgin olive oil

I red bell pepper, small dice

3 tablespoons diced red onion

½ medium zucchini, small dice

½ medium yellow squash, small dice

6 egg whites

6 whole eggs

¼ teaspoon dried thyme

½ teaspoon salt-free onion & herb seasoning

4 ounces fat-free cheddar cheese, to be split between 12 muffins

I cup of strawberries, sliced, on the side

Heat the olive oil over medium-high heat in a nonstick skillet.

Once oil is hot, add bell peppers, onions, zucchini, and squash. Sauté until the vegetables are soft and have a light brown color. Set aside and allow them to cool.

Meanwhile, whisk together egg whites and whole eggs along with dried thyme and onion herb seasoning.

Generously spray muffin pan with cooking spray to prevent sticking. Preheat oven to 400 degrees.

Distribute 1½ tablespoons of vegetable mixture into each muffin cup. Then evenly divide fat-free cheddar cheese between all 12 muffins.

Add egg mixture so that each cup is ¾ full.

Bake in preheated oven for approximately 20 minutes or until tops are light brown and the eggs are cooked through. Enjoy muffins with strawberries on the side.

Makes 12 muffins

Women (3 muffins): 285 cals; 15g fat; 17g carb; 24g protein
Men (4 muffins): 360 cals; 20g fat; 19g carb; 32g protein

Cinnamon French Toast

Breakfast

I whole egg (2 eggs for men)

I tablespoon unsweetened almond milk

Dash of cinnamon

2 slices low-sodium Ezekiel Sprouted
Grain Bread

¼ cup low-fat cottage cheese (½ cup for
men) (low sodium)

Vanilla stevia drops for sweetness

¼ cup berries

2 tablespoons sugar-free syrup

Spray a pan or skillet with cooking spray and place on medium heat.

Beat the egg, almond milk, and cinnamon together in a shallow dish. Dip both slices of the bread into the mixture, coating both sides. Place on the skillet and cook until the bread is brown on both sides.

Mix together the cottage cheese and stevia drops. Top French toast with sweetened cottage cheese, berries, and syrup. Enjoy!

Women: 295 cals; 6g fat; 39g carb; 21g protein
Men: 400 cals; 11g fat; 42g carb; 33g protein

Egg and Cheddar Sandwich

Breakfast

5 ounces sweet potato, cut into 4 rounds
(6 ounces for men)

2 whole eggs (3 eggs + 1 egg white for
men)

½ slice cheddar cheese

½ cup spinach

Preheat oven to 425 degrees. Spray baking sheet with cooking spray. Slice the sweet potato and place it on a greased baking sheet. Bake 20 minutes, then flip. Bake another 20 minutes.

Spray a frying pan with cooking spray and fry the eggs over medium-high heat until cooked through. Cut the fried eggs in half, and then fold in half.

Make 2 sandwiches by layering a sweet potato round, fried egg, ½ of the cheese and spinach, and another sweet potato round.

Women: 310 cals; 11g fat; 30g carb; 17g protein
Men: 420 cals; 15g fat; 36g carb; 27g protein

Green Machine Pancakes

Breakfast

2 whole eggs (3 eggs for men)

¼ cup low-fat cottage cheese

¼ cup rolled oats (⅓ cup for men)

½ banana

½ cup of spinach (I cup for men)

I tablespoon sugar-free syrup

Spray skillet or griddle with cooking spray and preheat to 300 degrees.

Place all ingredients except syrup in a blender and blend until smooth.

Pour the batter slowly onto griddle. Once bubbles form on top of pancake, flip. Top with sugar-free syrup.

Makes about 6 pancakes

Women: 315 cals; 11g fat; 30g carb; 22g protein
Men: 411 cals; 16g fat; 35g carb; 29g protein

Hot Quinoa Cereal with Banana

Breakfast

½ cup unsweetened vanilla almond milk

½ teaspoon Truvia sweetener

¼ teaspoon ground cinnamon

Pinch of ground nutmeg

½ cup cooked quinoa

½ scoop vanilla protein powder (I scoop for men)

½ banana, sliced (I full banana for men)

I tablespoon Pumpkin Seed Granola (page 212)

In a small pot bring almond milk, Truvia, cinnamon, and nutmeg to a light simmer.

Add cooked quinoa and stir. Then add the scoop of protein powder and stir until protein is thoroughly dissolved.

Transfer to a bowl and top with sliced banana and granola.

Women: 300 cals; 9g fat; 37g carb; 20g protein
Men: 420 cals; 10g fat; 52g carb; 34g protein

Huevos Rancheros

Breakfast

Egg Scramble

1 teaspoon extra-virgin olive oil (2 teaspoons for men)

½ cup red bell pepper, diced

½ cup green bell pepper, diced

¼ cup red onion, diced

4 egg whites (6 egg whites for men)

Pinch of black pepper

Pinch of salt-free southwest seasoning

1 tablespoon low-fat mozzarella cheese (2 tablespoons for men)

2 tablespoons fresh salsa

In a nonstick skillet, heat the extra-virgin olive oil and lightly sauté the peppers and onions. Once the vegetables are soft, add egg whites, black pepper, and southwest seasoning.

Scramble the egg mixture until egg whites are fully cooked. Serve over tostadas. Top with cheese and fresh salsa.

Tostadas

2 yellow corn tortillas

Lightly spray tortilla with cooking spray and bake in a 425-degree oven until golden brown and crispy.

Women: 300 cals; 8g fat; 35g carb; 21g protein

Men: 390 cals; 15g fat; 36g carb; 30g protein

"Loaded" Breakfast Potato

Breakfast

6 tablespoons fat-free plain Greek yogurt
(¾ cup for men)

Truvia sweetener

Pinch of ground cinnamon

1 tablespoon unsalted almond butter

¼ cup quinoa, cooked

4 ounces (½ cup) cooked sweet potato
(6 ounces or ¾ cup for men)

In a small dish, mix the yogurt, Truvia, and cinnamon.

In a separate dish, mix the almond butter with the quinoa.

Slice the warm potato down the middle and spread it open. Top with the almond butter mixture and then top with cinnamon yogurt.

Women: 300 cals; 10g fat; 38g carb; 15g protein
Men: 400 cals; 10g fat; 52g carb; 25g protein

No-Bake Oats

Breakfast

⅓ cup rolled oats

¼ cup vanilla or chocolate protein powder (½ cup for men)

2 tablespoons powdered peanut butter

2 teaspoons ground flaxseed or chia
seeds

⅓ cup unsweetened almond milk

½ banana, sliced (⅔ banana for men)

Dash of cinnamon

Mix the oats, protein powder, powdered peanut butter, and flax or chia seeds. Add the almond milk. Stir. Top with banana slices and a dash of cinnamon.

Women: 300 cals; 8g fat; 40g carb; 24g protein
Men: 400 cals; 10g fat; 47g carb; 38g protein

Power Mocha Shake with Fruit

Breakfast

8 ounces black coffee, room temperature

1 scoop chocolate protein powder (1½ scoops for men)

¼ teaspoon ground cinnamon

½ tablespoon coconut oil

6–8 ice cubes (or 1 cup)

Blend everything in a blender until smooth. Enjoy with a side of sliced fruit: 1 banana (1½ bananas for men) or 1 cup berries (1½ cups for men).

Women: 300 cals; 10g fat; 28g carb; 28g protein
Men: 370 cals; 11g fat; 30g carb; 41g protein

Pumpkin Spice Vanilla Protein Pancakes

Breakfast

½ scoop vanilla protein powder (¾ scoop for men)

¼ cup pumpkin puree

1 teaspoon coconut oil

½ teaspoon ground cinnamon

¼ teaspoon ground nutmeg

½ teaspoon baking powder

1 large egg white

¼ cup steel-cut oats

⅓ cup water

1 teaspoon Truvia sweetener

¼ cup sugar-free pancake syrup

½ tablespoon Pumpkin Seed Granola (page 212)

½ banana, sliced (men only)

Add all ingredients except syrup, granola, and banana to the blender and blend until smooth.

Heat a nonstick griddle or skillet coated with cooking spray over medium heat. Ladle about ¼ cup of pancake batter per pancake onto griddle or skillet. Once pancake tops are covered with bubbles and edges look cooked, they are ready to flip. Cook both sides. Serve immediately. Top with syrup, granola, and banana (for men).

Makes 4 pancakes

Women: 310 cals; 11g fat; 34g carb; 25g protein
Men: 400 cals; 12g fat; 48g carb; 32g protein

Raspberry Almond Oatmeal

Breakfast

⅓ cup rolled oats (½ cup for men)

½ cup water

2 teaspoons all-natural almond butter

1 tablespoon unsweetened almond milk (2 tablespoons for men)

⅛ teaspoon pure almond extract (optional)

¼ cup vanilla protein powder (½ cup for men)

½ cup raspberries

1 teaspoon slivered almonds

Dash of cinnamon

Vanilla stevia drops for sweetness

Mix the oats and water together. Microwave 1–2 minutes.

Stir in almond butter, almond milk, and almond extract (if using). Stir in protein powder. Top with raspberries, almonds, and cinnamon. Add stevia if needed for sweetness. Eat warm.

You can also make this the night before by mixing all the ingredients together and storing in the fridge overnight without cooking. Eat cold.

Women: 285 cals; 11g fat; 30g carb; 20g protein
Men: 405 cals; 14g fat; 41g carb; 35g protein

Scrambled Eggs and Hash

Breakfast

½ cup mushrooms, sliced (1 cup for men)

¼ cup yellow onions, diced

4 ounces red potatoes, grated (5 ounces for men)

1 cup spinach, chopped

2 whole eggs (3 eggs + 1 egg white for men)

2 tablespoons fresh salsa

Heat pan or skillet to medium-high heat.

Spray pan with cooking spray. Sauté the mushrooms, onions, and potatoes together for 5 minutes. Add the spinach and eggs. Cook until the eggs are cooked through. Top with salsa.

Women: 293 cals; 10g fat; 27g carb; 18g protein
Men: 414 cals; 15g fat; 33g carb; 29g protein

Sweet Potato Fritters

Breakfast

1 ounce ground beef, browned (2 ounces for men)

2 tablespoons yellow onions, browned

2 whole eggs

3 ounces sweet potatoes, grated (4 ounces for men)

Salt-free garlic & herb seasoning

Black pepper

2 tablespoons low-fat mozzarella cheese

Preheat oven to 350 degrees.

Brown the ground beef with the onions. Set aside.

Beat the eggs. Add the ground beef, sweet potatoes, and seasonings. Mix well.

Spoon mixture into 2–3 well-greased muffin cups. Bake for 20 minutes. Pull out and sprinkle with cheese. Bake an additional 5–10 minutes.

Women: 300 cals; 14g fat; 20g carb; 21g protein
Men: 400 cals; 20g fat; 22g carb; 28g protein

Turkey and Potato Skillet Breakfast

Breakfast

1 teaspoon extra-virgin olive oil (2 teaspoons for men)

3 ounces extra-lean ground turkey breast (4 ounces for men)

½ red bell pepper, large dice

½ green bell pepper, large dice

¼ red onion, large dice

¼ teaspoon salt-free garlic & herb seasoning

Pinch of whole fennel seed

Pinch of dried oregano

Pinch of dried basil

Pinch of salt substitute

Pinch of ground black pepper

3 small sage leaves, fresh, chopped

½ cup cooked sweet potatoes, diced (¾ cup for men)

Heat olive oil in a nonstick skillet over medium heat.

Crumble ground turkey into skillet and stir to prevent sticking.

Add bell peppers and onions and cook until soft. Add garlic and herb seasoning, fennel seed, oregano, basil, salt substitute, black pepper, and sage. Stir to mix thoroughly.

Add sweet potatoes and cook until potatoes are heated through and have slight golden color.

Women: 275 cals; 6g fat; 32g carb; 23g protein
Men: 390 cals; 11g fat; 42g carb; 31g protein

Turkey Frittata

Breakfast

1 ounce extra-lean ground turkey

⅔ cup grated sweet potatoes (1 cup for men)

¼ teaspoon dried oregano

¼ teaspoon dried basil

Pinch of salt substitute

Pinch of ground black pepper

Pinch of whole fennel seeds

1 tablespoon diced onion

2 small mushrooms, sliced

1 whole egg

1 egg white (3 whites for men)

2 tablespoons shredded mozzarella cheese

3 cherry tomatoes, halved

¼ cup parsley leaves, rinsed

Lightly spray cooking spray over the grated potatoes and microwave 2 minutes.

Heat a nonstick frying pan over medium-high heat. Spray with cooking spray and crumble in ground turkey. Once turkey has a slight brown color, add oregano, basil, salt substitute, black pepper, fennel seeds, diced onions, and sliced mushrooms.

Cook mixture until vegetables are soft and turkey is fully cooked.

Add eggs and cheese. Cover and cook until eggs are cooked through.

Toss halved cherry tomatoes and parsley and place on top.

Women: 292 cals; 8g fat; 31g carb; 24g protein
Men: 385 cals; 8g fat; 44g carb; 32g protein

HIGH-CARB MEALS

Apple and Dip

High-Carb Meal

3 tablespoons fat-free plain Greek yogurt
(6 tablespoons for men)

½ scoop vanilla protein powder
(1 scoop for men)

2 tablespoons powdered peanut butter

Dash of cinnamon

1 medium apple (1 large apple for men)

Stevia, to taste

Mix yogurt, protein powder, peanut butter powder, stevia, and cinnamon.
Slice apple and dip!

Women: 240 cals; 3g fat; 34g carb; 24g protein
Men: 355 cals; 4g fat; 43g carb; 42g protein

Barbecue Chicken Salad

High-Carb Meal

Salad

1 ounce chicken breast, cooked and
cubed (3 ounces for men)

1 tablespoon low-sodium barbecue sauce
(3 tablespoons for men)

2 cups romaine lettuce, chopped

½ tomato, diced

¼ cup black beans

¼ cup fresh corn

Mix barbecue sauce with chicken, set aside.
Make salad by layering lettuce, tomatoes, beans, corn, and chicken.

Cilantro Lime Dressing

¼ cup fat-free plain Greek yogurt
1 tablespoon Homemade Ranch Powder
(see recipe below)

Pinch of cilantro
1 teaspoon lime juice
1 tablespoon low-sodium barbecue sauce

Make dressing by blending Greek yogurt, Ranch Powder, cilantro, and lime juice together. This recipe makes a lot of dressing; add to salad a tablespoon at a time. Top with remaining 1 tablespoon barbecue sauce.

Homemade Ranch Powder

½ cup dried buttermilk
1 tablespoon dried parsley flakes
1 teaspoon dried dill weed
1 teaspoon dried minced onion

1 teaspoon onion powder
½ teaspoon garlic powder
¼ teaspoon ground black pepper

In a small bowl, whisk all ingredients until combined.

Women: 260 cals; 5g fat; 44g carb; 24g protein
Men: 370 cals; 7g fat; 48g carb; 41g protein

BBQ Baked Sweet Potato, Loaded with Grilled Chicken, Corn, and Black Beans

High-Carb Meal

½ cup baked sweet potato (¾ cup for men)
2 ounces grilled diced chicken (3 ounces for men)
2 tablespoons frozen corn, thawed
¼ cup cooked black beans

1 tablespoon reduced-sugar barbecue sauce
Pinch of black pepper
Pinch of salt substitute
¼ cup chopped steamed broccoli

Poke holes in the sweet potato and bake it in the oven at 400 degrees for 45 minutes or for 8 minutes in the microwave.

In a mixing bowl, mix the grilled chicken, thawed corn, cooked black beans, and barbecue sauce and season with black pepper and salt subtitute. Stir until all ingredients have been evenly coated with sauce. Spoon the mixture into the middle of the sweet potato. Place the broccoli on top of the chicken mixture.

Women: 290 cals; 5g fat; 44g carb; 25g protein
Men: 385 cals; 6g fat; 54g carb; 35g protein

Butternut Squash Chili

High-Carb Meal

8 ounces extra-lean ground turkey

Cooking spray

2 cups peeled and cubed butternut squash

½ cup red onion, medium dice

2 tablespoons garlic, minced

½ cup red bell pepper, medium dice

½ cup green bell pepper, medium dice

½ medium jalapeño, stems and seeds removed (add more for extra heat)

2 tablespoons ground cumin

1 tablespoon light chili powder

½ tablespoon salt substitute

1 tablespoon smoked paprika

½ tablespoon ground mustard

1 quart water

1½ cups diced tomatoes in the can, no salt

4 tablespoons tomato paste

¼ cup apple cider vinegar

½ cup cooked black beans, no salt

½ cup cooked garbanzo beans, no salt

½ cup cilantro, rinsed and chopped

½ cup edamame, shelled

Brown the ground turkey and set aside. Spray a large pot with cooking spray, then over medium-high heat. Add the squash and stir until the squash has a light caramelized color.

Add the onions, garlic, red bell pepper, green bell pepper, and jalapeño. Stir and cook until the onions are translucent and the peppers are semi-soft.

Add the browned ground turkey, cumin, chili powder, salt substitute, paprika, mustard, water, canned tomatoes, tomato paste, and vinegar.

Simmer chili on medium-low for about 25 minutes or until the squash is tender.

Add the black beans, garbanzo beans, cilantro, and edamame. Stir to incorporate beans. Separate into 3 servings.

Note: This chili recipe is a Powell Pack favorite, so here's a three-serving recipe so there's enough to go around. If you're cooking for one, be sure to measure out your portion, then store and refrigerate the rest for healthy meals over the next few days.

Makes 3 servings

Women (1 serving): 294 cals; 3g fat; 39g carb; 29g protein
Men (1⅓ servings): 392 cals; 4g fat; 52g carb; 38g protein

Chicken Fajita Bowl

High-Carb Meal

½ cup onions, chopped

½ cup bell peppers, chopped

¼ cup brown rice, cooked (⅓ cup for men)

2 ounces chicken breast, cooked and cubed (4 ounces for men)

2 tablespoons black beans (¼ cup for men)

1 tablespoon low-fat mozzarella cheese

2 tablespoons fresh salsa

1 tablespoon fat-free plain Greek yogurt

Slice the onions into rings and the peppers into thin strips. Spray a frying pan or skillet with cooking spray and sauté until peppers are tender and onions are translucent.

Layer the rice, chicken, onions, peppers, black beans, cheese, salsa, and Greek yogurt. Enjoy!

Women: 292 cals; 6g fat; 38g carb; 26g protein
Men: 394 cals; 8g fat; 49g carb; 37g protein

Chile Relleno, Braised Adobo Chicken, Black Bean and Quinoa Salad

High-Carb Meal

Adobo Chicken

½ cup fresh salsa

½ teaspoon garlic, minced

2 tablespoons red onion, diced

¼ teaspoon salt-free southwest chipotle seasoning

½ teaspoon salt-free tomato basil seasoning

½ jalapeño, stems and seeds removed and finely diced

2 ounces grilled and diced marinated chicken (3 ounces chicken for men) (Marinade recipe below)

½ teaspoon fresh lime juice

2 teaspoons cilantro, rinsed and chopped

1 medium poblano pepper, dry roasted and peeled

In a skillet over medium heat, add the salsa, garlic, onion, southwest seasoning, tomato basil seasoning, and jalapeño. Bring to a simmer; add diced grilled chicken, lime juice, and cilantro.

Heat until chicken is hot all the way through.

Cut a slit in the pepper and stuff with chicken mixture. Microwave until hot. Serve over Black Bean and Quinoa Salad.

Marinade

3 sprigs fresh thyme or pinch of dried thyme

3 sprigs of fresh tarragon

1 tablespoon chopped garlic

1 tablespoon chopped yellow onion

2 tablespoons lemon juice

1 teaspoon salt-free chicken seasoning

½ teaspoon salt substitute

⅛ teaspoon black pepper

½ cup water

Place the thyme, tarragon, garlic, chopped onion, lemon juice, chicken seasoning, salt substitute, black pepper, and water in blender and blend until smooth.

Black Bean and Quinoa Salad

¼ cup cooked quinoa (½ cup for men)

¼ cup thawed corn

¼ cup cooked black beans

1 teaspoon salt-free garlic & herb seasoning

½ teaspoon salt-free southwest seasoning

½ teaspoon salt-free chicken seasoning

2 tablespoons fresh lime juice

Pinch of salt substitute

1 tablespoon cilantro, chopped and rinsed

Cook the quinoa and cool, toss with corn, black beans, garlic herb seasoning, southwest seasoning, chicken seasoning, fresh lime juice, salt substitute, and cilantro.

Women: 273 cals; 2g fat; 30g carb; 19g protein
Men: 349 cals; 5g fat; 40g carb; 26g protein

Chocolate Peanut Butter and Banana Smoothie

High-Carb Meal

1 frozen banana, chopped
½ scoop chocolate protein powder
  (1 scoop for men)
2 tablespoons chocolate peanut butter
  powder

1 tablespoon flax seeds
½ cup unsweetened vanilla almond milk
  (1 cup for men)
2 tablespoons rolled oats (men only)
6–8 ice cubes (or 1 cup)

Place all ingredients in a blender. Blend until smooth.

Women: 275 cals; 7g fat; 36g carb; 22g protein
Men: 400 cals; 11g fat; 46g carb; 37g protein

Egg Salad on Toast

High-Carb Meal

4 boiled egg whites (6 egg whites for
  men)
1 tablespoon low-fat mayo (2 tablespoons
  for men)
1 cup spinach

2 slices Ezekiel low-sodium bread,
  toasted
Paprika
Black pepper
½ cup blueberries (1 cup for men)

Boil eggs for 10–12 minutes. Place in ice water until cool. Peel eggs and separate yolk from white. Discard yolk.
   Mash egg whites and mayo together in a bowl.
   Layer ½ cup spinach on each piece of toast and top with egg salad. Sprinkle paprika and pepper over the top. Enjoy blueberries on the side.

Women: 290 cals; 3g fat; 44g carb; 24g protein
Men: 380 cals; 4g fat; 56g carb; 32g protein

Greek Yogurt Parfait with Fruit

High-Carb Meal

⅔ cup fat-free plain Greek yogurt
(1¼ cups for men)

Vanilla liquid stevia drops for sweetness
(optional)

½ cup sliced blackberries

½ cup strawberries, chopped

½ banana, sliced (1 banana for men)

Dash of cinnamon

Sweeten yogurt with stevia if desired. Top yogurt with blackberries, strawberries, bananas, and cinnamon.

Women: 290 cals; 4g fat; 36g carb; 20g protein
Men: 380 cals; 5g fat; 55g carb; 34g protein

Green Chili Turkey and Cilantro Rice Bowl

High-Carb Meal

Green Chili Turkey

3 ounces extra-lean ground turkey
(4 ounces for men)

1 red bell pepper, diced

¼ cup red onion, chopped

1 medium poblano pepper, roasted and
diced

1 small green tomatillo or green tomato

¼ teaspoon ground cumin

¼ teaspoon smoked paprika

¼ teaspoon dried oregano

Pinch of salt substitute

Pinch of ground black pepper

¼ cup water

Pinch of ground cayenne pepper

1 tablespoon cilantro, rinsed and chopped

Juice of ½ lime

Heat a skillet to medium-high heat. Spray with cooking spray. Crumble turkey into the skillet and stir to break up into small pieces.

Add bell peppers, red onion, roasted poblano, green tomatillo, cumin, paprika, oregano, salt substitute, black pepper, water, and cayenne. Stir and cook until turkey is cooked through.

Add cilantro and lime juice. Serve over Cilantro Rice.

Cilantro Rice

¼ cup cooked brown rice (½ cup for men)
I tablespoon chopped cilantro
½ tablespoon lime juice

Pinch of ground cumin
Pinch of salt substitute
Pinch of black pepper

Cook rice and toss with cilantro, lime juice, cumin, salt substitute, and black pepper.

Green Beans

I cup of green beans

Steam and toss with turkey mixture. Serve over Cilantro Rice.

Women: 305 cals; 3g fat; 44g carb; 27g protein
Men: 390 cals; 4g fat; 55g carb; 34g protein

Grilled Ginger Lime Tuna and Steamed Vegetable Medley

High-Carb Meal

Tuna

½ tablespoon rice vinegar, unseasoned
¾ teaspoon salt-free onion & herb seasoning
I tablespoon ginger, minced
¼ teaspoon Sriracha sauce

¼ teaspoon Truvia sweetener
Pinch of salt substitute
Pinch of ground black pepper
4 ounces wild tuna (6 ounces for men)
I lime wedge

In a medium mixing bowl, whisk together vinegar, onion and herb seasoning, minced ginger, Sriracha sauce, Truvia sweetener, salt substitute, ground black pepper, and juice from lime wedge until sweetener is dissolved. Once mixed, pour over tuna and spread evenly.

Marinate for at least one hour, being sure to rotate after 30 minutes.

Grill to preferred doneness, slice, and serve over rice and vegetables.

Vegetables

¾ cup snap peas

1½ ounces carrots, cut to preference

1 ounce chopped asparagus

½ cup steamed brown rice (1 cup for men)

Steam vegetables and toss together with rice.

Women: 268 cals; 5g fat; 22g carb; 27g protein
Men: 376 cals; 6g fat; 44g carb; 32g protein

Grilled Greek Chicken Kebabs

High-Carb Meal

Kebabs

2 ounces marinated chicken breast
(4 ounces for men)

Use Marinade recipe for chicken and then weigh and skewer chicken. Grill until chicken is cooked through. Serve potatoes and cauliflower on the side, and drizzle the kebabs and vegetables with yogurt sauce. The yogurt sauce can also be used as a dipping sauce.

Marinade

3 sprigs fresh thyme or pinch of dried thyme

3 sprigs fresh tarragon

1 tablespoon chopped garlic

1 tablespoon chopped yellow onion

2 tablespoons lemon juice

1 teaspoon salt-free chicken seasoning

½ teaspoon salt substitute

Black pepper, to taste

½ cup water

Place thyme, tarragon, garlic, chopped onion, lemon juice, chicken seasoning, salt substitute, black pepper, and water in blender and blend until smooth. Marinate chicken in mixture for 2–24 hours.

Roasted Potatoes

1 cup red potatoes cut into wedges
    (1½ cups for men)
¼ teaspoon extra-virgin olive oil

1 sprig rosemary, chopped fine
Dash of salt substitute
Dash of ground black pepper

In a small pot, boil the potatoes in water until fork tender but not overcooked. Drain well and toss with extra-virgin olive oil.

In a skillet over high heat, lightly spray with cooking spray. Add potato wedges and stir frequently. Potatoes will get light brown in color. When this happens, add chopped rosemary, salt substitute, and ground black pepper. Stir well and remove from heat.

Yogurt Sauce

1 tablespoon fat-free plain Greek yogurt
1 tablespoon cucumber, small dice
4 small mint leaves, chopped
½ tablespoon green onion, chopped fine

½ teaspoon fresh lemon juice
Pinch of salt substitute
Pinch of black pepper

Mix all ingredients in a small bowl and allow to sit for 30 minutes before use. This will help the flavor develop better.

Cauliflower

4 ounces or 1 cup cauliflower "steak"—
    feel free to use florets already cut

¼ teaspoon salt-free onion & herb
    seasoning
¼ teaspoon olive oil

In a small skillet, cover cauliflower halfway with water and bring to a simmer. After 3 minutes, flip the cauliflower and let it simmer another 2 minutes. Remove from water and drain excess water.

In a small skillet, heat olive oil over medium-high heat. Season cauliflower on both sides with onion herb seasoning. Brown both sides of cauliflower, approximately 2 minutes on each side.

Women: 290 cals; 4g fat; 40g carb; 25g protein
Men: 410 cals; 5g fat; 56g carb; 36g protein

Homemade Tortilla Chips with Tomato Salsa

High-Carb Meal

Tortilla Chips

3 6-inch yellow corn tortillas (4 for men)
Pinch of cumin
Pinch of salt substitute

2 ounces shredded chicken (3 ounces for men)
½ cup Tomato Salsa (recipe below)

Cut the tortillas into wedges and lay them on a baking sheet lined with foil.

Preheat oven to 400 degrees. Lightly spray the tortillas with cooking spray and bake in the oven until crispy and golden brown.

Remove from the oven and sprinkle with cumin and salt substitute, then top with chicken and salsa.

Tomato Salsa

1 cup chopped fresh tomatoes
½ cup chopped red onion
¼ jalapeño, stem and seeds removed
10 sprigs cilantro, rinsed
1 tablespoon chopped garlic
2 tablespoons lime juice

1 teaspoon salt-free southwest seasoning
½ teaspoon salt substitute
½ teaspoon ground cumin
½ teaspoon light chili powder
¼ teaspoon ground black pepper

Place all ingredients in a blender and pulse until a salsa-like texture has been achieved.

Women: 290 cals; 4g fat; 40g carb; 22g protein
Men: 390 cals; 6g fat; 51g carb; 32g protein

Honey Dijon Chicken Snack Wrap

High-Carb Meal

2 ounces chicken breast, cooked and
   shredded (3 ounces for men)
1 Ezekiel tortilla (1½ tortillas for men)
1 cup baby spinach

½ cup sprouts
½ cup cucumbers, chopped
1 tablespoon honey Dijon mustard
Cracked pepper

Cook the chicken breast and shred it with two forks. Place it in the fridge to cool.
Pile all ingredients into the tortilla and roll up. Eat cold.

Women: 280 cals; 6g fat; 30g carb; 25g protein
Men: 400 cals; 9g fat; 42g carb; 37g protein

Hulk Shake

High-Carb Meal

4 ounces fresh orange juice (6 ounces for
   men)
2 cups power greens (spinach, chard, or
   kale)
⅔ cup fat-free plain Greek yogurt

¼ cup vanilla protein powder (men only)
1 frozen banana
Vanilla stevia drops for sweetness
6–8 ice cubes (or 1 cup)

Place all ingredients in a blender. Blend until smooth. Add water if needed to blend.

Women: 270 cals; 1g fat; 49g carb; 20g protein
Men: 365 cals; 2g fat; 57g carb; 34g protein

Italian Tuna and White Bean Lettuce Wraps

High-Carb Meal

2 ounces canned light white tuna, no salt added (4 ounces for men)

⅔ cup white beans, boiled, no salt (I cup for men)

¼ red bell pepper, diced

I teaspoon diced red onion

½ tablespoon parsley, chopped

¼ teaspoon salt-free tomato basil seasoning

I sprig fresh tarragon, chopped

I medium basil leaf, chopped

I radish, sliced thin

¼ cup diced tomatoes

I teaspoon balsamic vinegar

Pinch of salt substitute

Pinch of black pepper

I teaspoon fresh lemon juice

3 large lettuce leaves; Boston, Bibb, or red leaf work well (more lettuce can be used)

Drain tuna and transfer to a medium mixing bowl. Add white beans, red bell pepper, red onion, chopped parsley, tomato basil seasoning, tarragon, basil, radish, diced tomatoes, balsamic vinegar, salt substitute, black pepper, and fresh lemon juice. Toss to ensure ingredients are evenly distributed.

Distribute evenly and serve in 3 lettuce leaves.

Makes I serving.

Women: 260 cals; 2g fat; 36g carb; 27g protein
Men: 400 cals; 2g fat; 51g carb; 45g protein

Lemon Poppy Seed Protein Bites

High-Carb Meal

¾ cup oat flour (this can also be made by blending I cup of oats in a food processor)

3 scoops vanilla protein powder

½ teaspoon baking soda

2 teaspoons poppy seeds

4 egg whites

I cup unsweetened applesauce

2 tablespoons fat-free plain Greek yogurt

¼ cup lemon juice

I½ tablespoons lemon zest

2 teaspoons vanilla extract

Preheat the oven to 350 degrees. Prepare a 9 x 9-inch tin with cooking spray. In a small bowl, mix the oat flour, protein powder, baking soda, and poppy seeds.

In a separate bowl, mix together the egg whites, applesauce, yogurt, lemon juice, lemon zest, and vanilla extract.

Slowly add the dry ingredients to the wet ingredients and stir until everything is fully incorporated.

Pour mixture into sprayed pan and bake for about 30 minutes or until a toothpick comes out clean and the sides are light brown.

Remove from oven and allow to cool completely before cutting.

Note: Freeze leftovers and save for day 11.

Makes 12 evenly cut bars

Women (4 bars): 245 cals; 4g fat; 27g carb; 27g protein
Men (6 bars): 370 cals; 6g fat; 40g carb; 40g protein

Loaded Potato

High-Carb Meal

6 ounces red potato (8 ounces for men)

2 ounces extra-lean ground turkey, browned (4 ounces for men)

2 tablespoons yellow onions, browned

2 tablespoons shredded low-fat mozzarella cheese

2 tablespoons fat-free plain Greek yogurt (3 tablespoons for men)

2 teaspoons chives, chopped

½ tablespoon Homemade Ranch Powder (page 223)

Preheat oven to 400 degrees.

Poke holes in the potato with a fork. Wrap it in foil and bake for 45–60 minutes OR place in microwave-safe container and microwave for 8 minutes.

Brown turkey and onions together in a frying pan coated with cooking spray. Set aside.

Once potato is cooked, slice open and top with ground turkey and onions, cheese, yogurt, chives and Ranch Powder.

Women: 290 cals; 4g fat; 39g carb; 25g protein
Men: 400 cals; 5g fat; 49g carb; 41g protein

PB & J Rice Cakes and Shake

High-Carb Meal

Rice Cakes

3 tablespoons powdered peanut butter

2 tablespoons water

2 rice cakes, lightly salted (3 rice cakes for men)

Berry Puree (recipe below)

Mix powdered peanut butter and water together to reach a smooth consistency. Spread on each rice cake and top with Berry Puree. Enjoy with a protein shake.

Berry Puree

1 cup blackberries, washed (or any berry of choice)

2 tablespoons applesauce, unsweetened

1 tablespoon Truvia sweetener

In a blender, mix all ingredients on low until fully blended.

Shake

1 cup cold water or almond milk

½ scoop protein powder (1 scoop for men)

In a blender, mix ingredients on low until fully blended.

Women: 280 cals; 5g fat; 41g carb; 25g protein

Men: 385 cals; 6g fat; 50g carb; 39g protein

Peanut Butter Shake

High-Carb Meal

I cup unsweetened almond milk

¼ cup vanilla protein powder (½ cup for men)

2 tablespoons powdered peanut butter (¼ cup for men)

I frozen banana

6 ice cubes (or I cup)

Place all ingredients in a blender. Blend until smooth.

Women: 260 cals; 7g fat; 36g carb; 21g protein
Men: 375 cals; 9g fat; 42g carb; 39g protein

Piña Colada Dream

High-Carb Meal

¾ cup fat-free plain Greek yogurt (1½ cups for men)

Vanilla stevia drops for sweetness

⅛ teaspoon coconut extract (optional)

1½ cups fresh pineapple chunks (2 cups for men)

2 tablespoons reduced fat, unsweetened, finely shredded coconut

Stir the Greek yogurt, stevia, and coconut extract (if using) together in a bowl. Top with pineapple and shredded coconut.

Women: 265 cals; 3g fat; 42g carb; 20g protein
Men: 410 cals; 3g fat; 60g carb; 38g protein

Spiced Banana Shake

High-Carb Meal

½ cup unsweetened almond milk (1 cup for men)

1 frozen banana (1⅓ banana for men)

½ cup fat-free plain Greek yogurt

¼ cup vanilla protein powder (½ cup for men)

¼ teaspoon pure vanilla extract

Dash of nutmeg

Dash of cinnamon

20 liquid stevia drops

6 ice cubes

Place all ingredients in a blender. Blend until smooth.

Women: 275 cals; 4g fat; 35g carb; 27g protein
Men: 400 cals; 7g fat; 47g carb; 42g protein

Strawberry and Banana Quinoa Muffins

High-Carb Meal

1 cup white whole-wheat flour

1 teaspoon baking powder

½ teaspoon salt substitute

2 scoops vanilla protein powder

2 large eggs, beaten

1 teaspoon vanilla extract

1 tablespoon Truvia sweetener

2 tablespoons coconut oil, melted

2 medium bananas, mashed

1 cup chopped strawberries

1 cup cooked quinoa

Preheat the oven to 375 degrees. Prepare muffin or cupcake tins with cooking spray. In a small bowl, mix the flour, baking powder, salt substitute, and protein powder.

In a separate bowl, mix together eggs, vanilla, Truvia, and coconut oil.

Slowly add the dry ingredients to the wet ingredients and stir until everything is fully incorporated.

Fold in mashed bananas, strawberries, and cooked quinoa. Stir until evenly distributed.

Divide the batter among 12 muffin cups. Bake for about 25–30 minutes or until toothpick comes out clean when tested.

Note: Freeze leftovers and save for Day 17.

Makes 12 muffins

Women (2 muffins): 260 cals; 8g fat; 33g carb; 16g protein
Men (3 muffins): 385 cals; 12g fat; 50g carb; 23g protein

Sweet Potato Chips, Celery Sticks, and Shake

High-Carb Meal

1 cup sweet potato (1½ cups for men)
¼ teaspoon ground cumin
¼ teaspoon smoked paprika
¼ teaspoon garlic powder
¼ teaspoon dried basil

Pinch of light chili powder
Pinch of salt substitute
Pinch of ground black pepper
5 celery sticks
Cooking spray (fat-free)

Slice the sweet potatoes about ¼ inch thick and place them in a mixing bowl.

Lightly spray the sweet potatoes with cooking spray and ensure all sides are evenly coated.

Add the spices and toss until the sweet potatoes are evenly coated with spices.

Preheat oven to 275 degrees. Lay each sweet potato slice on a baking sheet lined with aluminum foil and place in oven.

Cook sweet potato slices for 15 minutes and then flip each one. Cook another 10 minutes and flip again. Cook for another 5 minutes or until potatoes are light brown and crispy.

Enjoy with the celery sticks and protein shake (recipe follows).

Shake

1 cup unsweetened almond milk
1 scoop protein powder (1½ scoops for men)

½ cup cold water (men only)
1 cup ice (optional)

Place all ingredients in a blender. Blend until smooth.

Women: 274 cals; 4g fat; 32g carb; 27g protein
Men: 391 cals; 4.6g fat; 47g carb; 40g protein

Sweet Wrap

High-Carb Meal

3 tablespoons fat-free plain Greek yogurt (¼ cup for men)

½ scoop vanilla protein powder (¾ scoop for men)

1 tablespoon powdered peanut butter (optional)

Vanilla stevia drops for sweetness (optional)

1 Rudi's spelt tortilla

½ banana, sliced (1 banana for men)

Dash of cinnamon

Mix Greek yogurt, powdered peanut butter, protein powder, and stevia together in a small bowl. Lay tortilla out on a plate; spread the yogurt mixture evenly down the center. Top with banana slices and cinnamon and wrap.

Women: 300 cals; 5g fat; 43g carb; 23g protein
Men: 410 cals; 6g fat; 60g carb; 32g protein

Three-Bean Salad with Chicken and Kale

High-Carb Meal

Salad

3 ounces grilled and diced marinated chicken (see Marinade recipe for Chile Relleno, page 225)

½ cup steamed and cut green beans

¼ cup garbanzo beans, boiled, no salt (½ cup for men)

¼ cup black beans, boiled, no salt (½ cup for men)

¼ cup boiled yellow beets

1 ounce shredded carrots

1 cup kale, washed well and shredded

In a medium mixing bowl, toss the grilled chicken, steamed green beans, garbanzo beans, black beans, beets, shredded carrots, and shredded kale. Mix with dressing (recipe follows).

Creamy Dressing

1 tablespoon fat-free plain Greek yogurt

1 tablespoon apple cider vinegar

Juice of ½ lemon

1 teaspoon salt-free tomato & garlic
    seasoning

1 teaspoon chopped parsley

Pinch of salt substitute

Pinch of ground black pepper

In a small mixing bowl, blend the yogurt, apple cider vinegar, lemon juice, tomato and garlic seasoning, chopped parsley, salt substitute, and black pepper until all ingredients are evenly distributed.

Women: 286 cals; 4g fat; 20g carb; 27g protein
Men: 412 cals; 5g fat; 37g carb; 31g protein

Triple Berry Treat

High-Carb Meal

⅔ cup fat-free cottage cheese (1¼ cups
    for men)

Vanilla stevia drops for sweetness

½ cup raspberries (⅔ cup for men)

½ cup blackberries (⅔ cup for men)

½ cup blueberries (⅔ cup for men)

½ cup Kashi GoLean Crisp cereal

Dash of cinnamon

Stir (or blend in a blender to make smooth) cottage cheese and stevia drops together until you reach your desired sweetness. Add berries, cereal, and cinnamon.

Women: 270 cals; 1g fat; 45g carb; 25g protein
Men: 385 cals; 2g fat; 58g carb; 40g protein

Turkey Sliders with Sweet Potato "Bun"

High-Carb Meal

6 ounces sweet potato (8 ounces for men)

3 ounces extra-lean ground turkey (4 ounces for men)

Dash each of paprika, black pepper, garlic powder, and onion powder

2 tablespoons low-fat mozzarella cheese (3 tablespoons for men)

2 tomato slices

Spinach

1 teaspoon Dijon mustard (2 teaspoons for men)

Preheat oven to 425 degrees.

Cut the sweet potato into 4 rounds the size of a slider bun. Bake for 15 minutes. Remove from oven, flip, and then cook 15 more minutes.

Mix the ground turkey and seasonings together. Form turkey into 2 small patties. Grill or brown on a skillet. Once fully cooked, sprinkle cheese on top.

Use the sweet potato rounds for a bun and top burger with tomatoes, spinach, and mustard.

Makes 1 slider (2 for men)

Women: 290 cals; 3g fat; 36g carb; 25g protein
Men: 395 cals; 5g fat; 47g carb; 34g protein

LOW-CARB MEALS

Almond-Crusted Tilapia with Asparagus and Cauliflower Mash

Low-Carb Meal

Tilapia

½ teaspoon fat-free plain Greek yogurt

4 ounces tilapia filet (5 ounces for men)

¼ teaspoon salt-free garlic & herb seasoning

1 tablespoon Almond Crust (recipe below) (2 tablespoons for men)

¼ cup water

½ cup steamed asparagus

Spread yogurt evenly on top of tilapia. Top with garlic herb seasoning and Almond Crust. In a small nonstick skillet, add ¼ cup of water and bring to a simmer.

Carefully add the fish and simmer until the water evaporates. Once water evaporates, place the skillet in a preheated oven on high broil. Broil fish on high until crust is crispy and golden brown.

Serve with steamed asparagus, Cauliflower Mash, and Greek Yogurt Tartar Sauce.

Almond Crust

1 cooked tostada, broken into medium pieces

¼ cup sliced raw almonds

1 teaspoon smoked paprika

Pinch salt substitute

Pinch black pepper

Place all ingredients in a blender and blend until chopped fine.

Makes 8 servings, 1 tablespoon each

Cauliflower Mash

¼ head fresh cauliflower, cut into small, even pieces

1 tablespoon unsweetened almond milk

1 tablespoon fat-free plain Greek yogurt

2 teaspoons olive oil

Pinch of granulated garlic

Pinch of black pepper

Pinch of salt substitute

Pinch of chopped green onions

In a small pot, cover the cauliflower with water and bring to a boil. Cook for about 6 minutes or until it is fork tender.

Drain the cauliflower very well and shake off excess water.

Transfer the cooked cauliflower to a blender, food processer, or a mixing bowl with a hand masher. Add almond milk, yogurt, olive oil, garlic, pepper, salt substitute, and chopped green onions and mash well.

Greek Yogurt Tartar Sauce

¼ cup fat-free plain Greek yogurt

¼ cup cucumber, diced fine

1 tablespoon red onion, diced fine

½ teaspoon fresh lemon juice

1 teaspoon yellow mustard

¼ teaspoon apple cider vinegar

Pinch of black pepper

Pinch of garlic powder

Pinch of paprika

Pinch of Truvia sweetener

In a mixing bowl, mix all ingredients until evenly incorporated.

Makes 2 servings for men and 3 servings for women

Women: 290 cals; 17.5g fat; 4g carb; 30g protein
Men: 341 cals; 22.5g fat; 6g carb; 36g protein

Barbecue Grill Pork Tenderloin

Low-Carb Meal

Pork Tenderloin

¼ teaspoon black pepper

¼ teaspoon ground mustard powder

¼ teaspoon ground cumin

¼ teaspoon smoked paprika

¼ teaspoon garlic powder

¼ teaspoon onion powder

¼ teaspoon salt-free onion & herb seasoning

3 ounces lean pork tenderloin (5 ounces for men)

In a small bowl, mix pepper, mustard powder, cumin, paprika, garlic powder, onion powder, and onion and herb seasoning.

Rub pork generously with spice rub and marinate for 1 hour before cooking.

On a preheated grill, cook pork until it reaches 145 degrees. Let it cool for about 5 minutes before slicing. This will help keep it juicy.

Olive Oil Roasted Green Beans

¼ cup water

1 cup fresh green beans, clipped and trimmed

1 tablespoon extra-virgin olive oil

¼ tablespoon fresh rosemary, chopped fine

Pinch of dried thyme

Pinch of black pepper

Pinch of salt substitute

1 tablespoon sliced raw almonds, unsalted (men only)

In a nonstick skillet over medium-high heat, bring water to a simmer.

Add green beans and cook until water evaporates.

Once water evaporates, add olive oil, rosemary, thyme, pepper, and salt substitute.

Turn heat up to high and stir until green beans have a nice golden brown color. Add sliced almonds for men's version only.

Women: 280 cals; 17g fat; 8g carb; 24g protein
Men: 400 cals; 23g fat; 9g carb; 41g protein

Cajun Salmon with Cabbage Salad and Steamed Broccoli

Low-Carb Meal

Cajun Salmon

¼ teaspoon black pepper

¼ teaspoon ground mustard powder

¼ teaspoon ground cumin

¼ teaspoon smoked paprika

¼ teaspoon garlic powder

¼ teaspoon onion powder

Pinch of cayenne pepper

¼ teaspoon salt-free onion & herb seasoning

4 ounces wild caught salmon (5 ounces for men)

1 cup steamed broccoli

In a small bowl mix pepper, mustard, cumin, paprika, garlic powder, onion powder, cayenne pepper, and onion and herb seasoning.

Rub salmon generously with spice rub and let marinate for an hour before cooking.

Heat grill to medium heat. Lightly spray salmon with cooking spray, place on a piece of foil, and grill 5 minutes on each side. Let cool for about 5 minutes before serving. This will help keep it juicy.

Serve with steamed broccoli and Cabbage Slaw.

Cabbage Slaw

1 cup shredded green and red cabbage

1 ounce shredded carrots

1 tablespoon parsley, rinsed and chopped

¼ teaspoon Truvia sweetener

2 teaspoons extra-virgin olive oil

Pinch of pepper

Pinch of salt substitute

1 tablespoon Pumpkin Seed Granola (page 212)

In a mixing bowl, toss the cabbage with carrots, parsley, Truvia, olive oil, pepper, salt substitute, and granola. Toss well and allow to marinate for 30 minutes before serving.

Women: 279 cals; 19g fat; 4g carb; 26g protein
Men: 312 cals; 22g fat; 5g carb; 28g protein

Cauli Mash and Meatballs

Low-Carb Meal

3 ounces extra-lean ground turkey, thawed (4 ounces for men)

2 tablespoons yellow onion, minced

1 tablespoon chives, chopped

1 tablespoon cilantro, chopped

¼ teaspoon garlic powder (½ teaspoon for men)

1½ cups cauliflower florets (2 cups for men)

1 tablespoon fat-free plain Greek yogurt (2 tablespoons for men)

1 tablespoon butter, unsalted (1½ tablespoons for men)

2 tablespoons low-fat mozzarella cheese

¼ teaspoon salt-free seasoning (½ teaspoon for men)

⅛ teaspoon ground pepper

Heat a skillet to medium heat.

With hands, mix together ground turkey, onion, chives, cilantro, and garlic powder.

Using a cookie scoop, form turkey into balls and place on a skillet sprayed with cooking spray. Cook 4 minutes and flip. Continue to cook and rotate until all sides are browned.

Boil cauliflower florets for 10 minutes. Drain and remove from heat. Add Greek yogurt, butter, cheese, and seasonings. Beat with hand mixer for 3–5 minutes or until smooth and creamy.

Place meatballs on mashed cauli and enjoy!

Women: 290 cals; 16g fat; 11g carb; 28g protein
Men: 390 cals; 22g fat; 14g carb; 37g protein

Cheesy Chicken and String Beans

Low-Carb Meal

2 cups French-cut string beans

2 ounces chicken breast, chopped (4 ounces for men)

½ tablespoon coconut oil (1 tablespoon for men)

1 Laughing Cow cheese wedge

Garlic and herb salt-free seasoning

Black pepper

Cook the green beans according to the package directions. Set aside.

Brown the chicken in a skillet with coconut oil over medium heat. Add the green beans. Add the cheese and seasonings. Stir until the cheese is melted.

Women: 260 cals; 11g fat; 14g carb; 25g protein
Men: 420 cals; 20g fat; 14g carb; 43g protein

Chicken Basil Spaghetti

Low-Carb Meal

1 cup spaghetti squash	2 tablespoons feta cheese crumbles
2 ounces chicken, cooked and cubed (4 ounces for men)	½ tablespoon olive oil
2 cherry tomatoes, halved (4 for men)	1 tablespoon fresh basil, chopped
2 tablespoons black olives	1 teaspoon dried minced onion
	Salt-free garlic & herb seasoning to taste

Preheat oven to 425 degrees.

Slice the spaghetti squash into 2-inch rings. Remove seeds and place on a baking sheet sprayed with cooking spray. Bake for 20 minutes. Flip. Bake an additional 20 minutes. Squash should be tender, but not mushy. Rake with a fork into a bowl.

Layer spaghetti squash, chicken, tomatoes, olives, and cheese. Top with olive oil, basil, onion, and garlic herb seasoning.

Women: 277 cals; 15g fat; 14g carb; 22g protein
Men: 376 cals; 17g fat; 16g carb; 40g protein

Chicken Slaw Dip

Low-Carb Meal

2 ounces chicken breast, cooked and shredded (4 ounces for men)	¼ teaspoon salt-free onion & herb seasoning
½ avocado, mashed	Black pepper
2 tablespoons fat-free plain Greek yogurt (¼ cup for men)	1 cup cabbage slaw
	1 cup cucumbers, sliced

Cook the chicken, shred it with two forks, and let cool in the fridge.

Combine the mashed avocado, Greek yogurt, and seasonings together. Add shredded chicken and slaw.

Dip the cucumbers in chicken slaw and eat cold.

Women: 260 cals; 13g fat; 14g carb; 23g protein
Men: 370 cals; 15g fat; 16g carb; 44g protein

Chipotle Turkey Burger with House Pickles

Low-Carb Meal

Turkey Burger

3 ounces extra lean ground turkey
(5 ounces for men)
Pinch of salt-free southwest seasoning
Pinch of black pepper
Pinch of dried thyme
Pinch of granulated garlic
Pinch of chili powder
Pinch of salt substitute

1 tablespoon red onion, small dice
1 small handful arugula or your preferred lettuce
¼ avocado, sliced (½ avocado, sliced, for men)
1 cup steamed broccoli
2 sliced tomatoes or cherry tomatoes halved

In a small bowl, mix the ground turkey, southwest seasoning, black pepper, thyme, garlic, chili powder, salt substitute, and red onion until evenly distributed. Make a patty. Lightly spray the grill with nonstick cooking spray, then cook on preheated grill until internal temperature reaches 165 degrees. Serve on top of arugula, top with avocado and serve with steamed broccoli, sliced tomatoes, and House Pickles (recipe follows).

House Pickles

¼ sliced cucumber
2 ounces Ginger Lime Sauce (see Vietnamese Grilled Chicken Spring Rolls, page 266)

¼ teaspoon Truvia sweetener
¼ teaspoon turmeric powder

Slice cucumbers as thinly as possible.
Mix together the Ginger Lime Sauce with Truvia and turmeric.
Toss cucumbers with sauce and refrigerate for at least 24 hours.

Women: 251 cals; 10.5g fat; 6g carb; 29g protein
Men: 331 cals; 17.5g fat; 7g carb; 31g protein

Chocolate Chip Almond Coconut Bites and Shake

Low-Carb Meal

Bites

½ cup oats

⅓ cup shredded and toasted coconut, unsweetened

¼ cup almond butter, no salt

2 tablespoons flax seeds

1 tablespoon dark chocolate chips

½ tablespoon coconut oil

½ tablespoon fat-free plain Greek yogurt

In a mixing bowl combine all ingredients until they are evenly distributed. Roll into 1-ounce balls; makes 6 bites. Store in the fridge or freezer in an airtight container. Enjoy 1 bite with a protein shake.

Protein Shake

1 cup unsweetened almond milk

¾ scoop protein powder (1½ scoops for men)

In a blender, mix all ingredients on low until fully blended.

Women (1 bite and shake): 280 cals; 16g fat; 12g carb; 24g protein
Men (1 bite and shake): 385 cals; 18g fat; 15g carb; 44g protein

Chocolate Peanut Butter Shake

Low-Carb Meal

I cup unsweetened almond milk

I scoop chocolate protein powder (1½ scoops for men)

I tablespoon all-natural peanut butter (1½ tablespoons for men)

6–8 ice cubes (or 1 cup)

Place all ingredients in a blender. Blend until smooth.

Women: 280 cals; 14g fat; 8g carb; 32g protein
Men: 400 cals; 19g fat; 11g carb; 47g protein

Citrus and Onion Fish Tacos

Low-Carb Meal

4 ounces white fish (mahi-mahi, tilapia, halibut, cod), thawed (6 ounces for men)

I tablespoon lime juice

I tablespoon apple cider vinegar

I teaspoon Truvia

½ teaspoon onion powder

½ avocado, diced (¾ avocado for men)

½ Roma tomato, diced

I tablespoon fat-free plain Greek yogurt (2 tablespoons for men)

2 tablespoons cilantro, chopped

½ lime, juiced

2 butter lettuce cups (3 for men)

Place the fish in a zip-lock bag with the tablespoon of lime juice, vinegar, Truvia, and onion powder and store in the fridge overnight.

Spray a pan with cooking spray. Pan-fry the fish with marinade over medium heat. Cook 5 minutes per side or until the fish flakes.

Layer the fish, avocado, tomatoes, Greek yogurt, cilantro, and lime juice evenly inside each butter lettuce cup. Enjoy!

Women: 265 cals; 12g fat; 18g carb; 25g protein
Men: 380 cals; 18g fat; 21g carb; 38g protein

Citrus Salmon Slaw

Low-Carb Meal

3 ounces wild caught salmon, cooked (5 ounces for men)

1 cup plain cabbage slaw (1½ cups for men)

2 asparagus spears, chopped

¼ cup sweet bell peppers

¼ avocado, sliced

2 tablespoons fat-free plain Greek yogurt (3 tablespoons for men)

2 tablespoons fresh salsa (3 tablespoons for men)

Cilantro

Lime juice

Salt-free garlic & herb seasoning, to taste

Spray a frying pan with cooking spray and pan-fry the salmon, 5 minutes on each side or until it flakes.

Layer the slaw, salmon, and veggies. Top with the yogurt, salsa, cilantro, and lime juice. Season with garlic and herb seasoning.

Women: 272 cals; 14g fat; 15g carb; 22g protein
Men: 394 cals; 20g fat; 20g carb; 34g protein

Creamy Cauliflower Soup

Low-Carb Meal

2 cups cauliflower, broken up

¼ cup yellow onion, chopped

1½ teaspoons olive oil

1 cup of low-sodium chicken broth

¼ teaspoon garlic, minced

⅓ cup fat-free plain Greek yogurt

⅓ cup low-fat mozzarella cheese

1 ounce chicken, cooked and shredded (3 ounces for men)

salt-free seasoning

Black pepper, to taste

Chives

Preheat oven to 375 degrees.

Place the cauliflower and onions in a baking dish, drizzle them with olive oil, and roast until golden, about 30 minutes.

Place the chicken broth and garlic in a pot and bring to a boil. Add the roasted cauliflower and onions. Boil for 5 minutes. Remove from heat. Add the Greek yogurt, cheese, and seasonings. Stir.

Puree in a blender or use a hand-held emulsifier to blend in the pot until smooth. Pour into a bowl and top with chives.

Women: 280 cals; 11g fat; 16g carb; 33g protein
Men: 390 cals; 15g fat; 16g carb; 52g protein

Curry Turkey Sliders with Cucumber and Tomato Salad

Low-Carb Meal

Sliders

4 ounces extra-lean ground turkey
   (6 ounces for men)
1 teaspoon ground yellow curry powder
1/3 teaspoon turmeric powder
1/2 teaspoon ground ginger
1/2 teaspoon ground black pepper

Pinch of garam masala
Pinch of ground coriander
Pinch of cayenne pepper
1 teaspoon cilantro, rinsed and chopped
   fine

In a large mixing bowl, mix all ingredients until everything is evenly distributed.

Once turkey is mixed, separate into 1-ounce balls and lightly press into thin patties. Lightly spray each turkey slider with cooking spray and place on a preheated grill. After about 2 minutes, flip to cook the other side.

Serve with Cucumber and Tomato Salad (recipe follows).

Cucumber and Tomato Salad

1 tablespoon fresh lime juice
1/2 tablespoon extra-virgin olive oil
1/4 tablespoon ground ginger
1/4 teaspoon ground black pepper
1/2 teaspoon Truvia sweetener
1 tablespoon fresh lemon juice

4 small mint leaves, chopped fine
1 medium cucumber, cubed
5 cherry tomatoes, halved
1/4 avocado (1/2 avocado for men)
2 tablespoons red onion, minced

In a mixing bowl whisk together lime juice, olive oil, ground ginger, black pepper, Truvia, lemon juice, and mint leaves. Whisk until seasonings have been dissolved.

Add cucumbers, cherry tomatoes, avocado, and red onion.
Toss all ingredients.

Women: 285 cals; 14g fat; 15g carb; 28g protein
Men: 400 cals; 20g fat; 17g carb; 42g protein

Deviled Eggs

Low-Carb Meal

3 whole eggs (4 eggs for men)

¼ cup fat-free plain Greek yogurt (men only)

1 tablespoon low-fat mayo

1 teaspoon Dijon mustard

Paprika

Black pepper

12 sugar snap peas (20 for men)

Boil eggs for 10–12 minutes. Put in ice water until cool. Peel and cut eggs in half.
Scoop all the yolks into a bowl. Mix yolks with Greek yogurt or mayo and mustard.
Fill each egg with the yolk mixture and top with a dash of paprika and pepper. Eat snap peas on the side.

Women: 250 cals; 13g fat; 5g carb; 19g protein
Men: 355 cals; 16g fat; 8g carb; 32g protein

Edamame and Pistachio Hummus with Cucumbers and Chicken

Low-Carb Meal

¾ cup water

½ cup raw edamame, shelled

½ tablespoon lemon juice

½ teaspoon garlic, chopped

2 tablespoons pistachios, raw and unsalted

⅛ teaspoon ground cumin

1 pinch of salt substitute

1 pinch of cayenne pepper

⅛ teaspoon ground black pepper

2 tablespoons extra-virgin olive oil

½ cucumber, sliced

2 ounces grilled chicken (4 ounces for men)

In a small pot, bring water to a boil and cook edamame for about 5 minutes or until fork tender. Once cooked, strain and reserve 2 tablespoons of the hot water for a later step.

Move strained edamame to a blender or food processor and add lemon juice, garlic, pistachios, cumin, salt substitute, cayenne, and black pepper. Pulsate to mix spices and coarsely blend the edamame.

With the blender going, slowly drizzle in the olive oil and then use the reserved water as needed to adjust the consistency.

Remove from blender and enjoy ½ cup hummus with sliced cucumbers and grilled chicken.

Makes 1 cup, or 2 servings

Women: 305 cals; 21g fat; 7g carb; 23g protein
Men: 400 cals; 23g fat; 7g carb; 41g protein

Eggplant Curry Stir-Fry

Low-Carb Meal

2 pieces firm tofu (4 pieces for men)
½ cup sliced yellow onions
½ medium eggplant, peeled and diced into 1-inch cubes
½ cup red bell pepper, diced
½ teaspoon cumin seed
½ teaspoon yellow mustard seed
¼ teaspoon ground turmeric
¼ teaspoon ground ginger
2 teaspoons curry powder
¼ teaspoon ground coriander
¼ teaspoon garam masala

¼ teaspoon red chili flakes
½ teaspoon salt substitute
¼ teaspoon black pepper
¼ teaspoon ground cumin
½ tablespoon Truvia sweetener
3 cups water
¼ cup lime juice
½ cup broccoli, raw and chopped
¼ cup shelled edamame
½ cup cilantro, chopped
1 tablespoon raw peanuts, unsalted, per serving

Spray a pan with cooking spray and add tofu, sliced onions, eggplant, bell peppers, cumin seed, and mustard seed. Cook this mixture until onions are golden brown, about 5–7 minutes.

Add turmeric, ginger, curry, coriander, garam masala, chili flakes, salt substitute, pepper, cumin, Truvia, and water. Bring to a simmer and cook until eggplant is tender.

Add lime juice, broccoli, edamame, and cilantro. Cook until broccoli is tender.

Serve 1 serving in a bowl with peanuts on top.

Makes 2 servings

Women: 285 cals; 13g fat; 25g carb; 21g protein
Men: 420 cals; 20g fat; 29g carb; 36g protein

Fajita Chicken Roll-Ups with Roasted Squash and Avocado Puree

Low-Carb Meal

Chicken Roll-Ups

¼ teaspoon salt-free southwest seasoning

¼ teaspoon salt-free onion & herb seasoning

¼ teaspoon salt-free chicken seasoning

Pinch of salt substitute

2 2-ounce chicken breasts, pounded thin (2 4-ounce breasts for men)

½ red bell pepper, cut into thin strips

½ red onion, cut into thin strips

In a small bowl, mix southwest seasoning, onion and herb seasoning, chicken seasoning, and salt substitute.

Lay the pounded chicken breasts out flat and evenly season with above mixture.

Mix peppers and onions and evenly distribute between the chicken breasts, ensuring the veggies are facing the same way. This will make rolling much easier.

Start by folding the closest part of the chicken over the vegetables and roll until vegetables are covered. Place seam down on a sheet tray and place in the freezer for about 20 minutes. This will help the cooking process.

Spray a nonstick skillet with cooking spray and heat over medium-high heat. Slowly add the chicken roll-ups with the open end first. Allow chicken to cook for about 4 minutes without moving. You want to create a nice seal so the roll-ups stay together. After about 4 minutes, roll the roll-ups over to cook the other side, about another 4 minutes or until internal temperature is 165 degrees. Serve with roasted squash and top with avocado puree.

Makes 2 servings

Roasted Zucchini and Squash

1 medium yellow squash, ½-inch dice
1 medium zucchini, ½-inch dice
¼ teaspoon dried thyme

¼ teaspoon red pepper flakes
¼ teaspoon black pepper

Heat a skillet on high heat. Spray with cooking spray and add squash and zucchini; stir immediately. Keep stirring until vegetables have a light brown color and are fork tender. Add seasonings and remove from heat.

Makes 2 servings

Avocado Puree

1 medium ripe avocado
1 tablespoon fresh lime juice
¼ teaspoon black pepper

¼ teaspoon ground cumin
Pinch of salt substitute

In a small bowl, cut avocado and smash with a spoon.
Add lime juice, pepper, cumin, and salt substitute. Mix with spoon until smooth.

Makes 4 servings for women and 2 for men

Women: 240 cals; 10g fat; 17g carb; 21g protein
Men: 415 cals; 19g fat; 21g carb; 39g protein

Greek Yogurt Parfait with Nuts

Low-Carb Meal

1 cup fat-free plain Greek yogurt
½ scoop vanilla protein powder (men only)
Vanilla stevia drops for sweetness (optional)

2 tablespoons sliced almonds, unsalted and raw
1 tablespoon chopped hazelnuts, unsalted and raw (2 tablespoons for men)

Sweeten yogurt with stevia if desired (men, stir in protein powder, too). Top with almonds and hazelnuts.

Women: 257 cals; 12g fat; 14g carb; 29g protein
Men: 360 cals; 17g fat; 16g carb; 42g protein

Grilled Lamb Kebabs

Low-Carb Meal

Lamb Kebabs

3 ounces lean lamb meat, preferably shoulder (5 ounces for men)

2 ounces All-Purpose Marinade (recipe below)

Cut lean lamb into 1-inch cubes, toss with marinade, and refrigerate for up to 24 hours. On a hot grill, cook to preferred doneness.

All-Purpose Marinade

3 sprigs fresh thyme or pinch of dried thyme

3 sprigs fresh tarragon

1 tablespoon chopped garlic

1 tablespoon chopped yellow onion

2 tablespoons lemon juice

1 teaspoon salt-free chicken seasoning

½ teaspoon salt substitute

Black pepper, to taste

½ cup water

Place thyme, tarragon, garlic, chopped onion, lemon juice, chicken seasoning, salt substitute, black pepper, and water in blender and blend until smooth.

Vegetables

1 teaspoon extra-virgin olive oil

3 ounces yellow squash, ½-inch dice

3 ounces zucchini, ½-inch dice

Pinch of dry thyme

Pinch of red pepper flakes

Pinch of black pepper

In a skillet over high heat, add olive oil and allow it to get hot. Add squash and zucchini and stir immediately. Keep stirring until vegetables have a light brown color and are fork tender. Add seasonings and remove from heat.

Women: 275 cals; 17g fat; 6g carb; 22g protein
Men: 405 cals; 25g fat; 6g carb; 36g protein

Grilled Wild Salmon with Quinoa and Edamame Salad

Low-Carb Meal

Fish

4 ounces wild caught salmon (6 ounces for men)

1 tablespoon salt-free onion & herb seasoning

Preheat grill to medium heat. Season the salmon with salt-free seasoning. Place salmon on foil and grill about 5 minutes per side or until desired doneness.

Salad

2 tablespoons cooked quinoa (¼ cup for men)

¼ cup edamame, shelled

2 asparagus spears, thinly chopped

½ tablespoon chopped parsley

½ teaspoon salt-free onion & herb seasoning

1 tablespoon fresh lemon juice

Dash of black pepper

Mix all ingredients together in a mixing bowl with a spatula. Serve with salmon.

Women: 280 cals; 13g fat; 12g carb; 27g protein
Men: 405 cals; 20g fat; 17g carb; 39g protein

Pepper Jack Chicken

Low-Carb Meal

3 ounces chicken breast, thawed (4½ ounces for men)

Salt-free seasoning

2 slices pepper jack cheese

8 asparagus spears (12 spears for men)

1 tablespoon Dijon mustard

Heat a skillet to medium heat.

Pound the chicken flat in between two sheets of parchment paper. Season with your favorite salt-free seasoning.

Place cheese on one side of the flattened chicken. Place asparagus stalks on top of cheese. Fold the other half of the chicken breast over the asparagus and cheese. Place the chicken in skillet. Cover. Cook 5 minutes on each side.

Top with mustard. Enjoy!

Women: 280 cals; 12g fat; 6g carb; 32g protein
Men: 383 cals; 16g fat; 9g carb; 47g protein

Popeye Shake

Low-Carb Meal

I cup frozen spinach

I tablespoon natural nut butter

½ cup unsweetened almond milk

I tablespoon milled flax (2 tablespoons for men)

I scoop protein powder (1½ scoops for men)

4–6 ice cubes (or ¾ cup)

Place all ingredients in a blender. Blend until smooth.

Women: 300 cals; 15g fat; 10g carb; 33g protein
Men: 405 cals; 19g fat; 14g carb; 48g protein

Protein Punch Wraps

Low-Carb Meal

1½ ounces chicken breast, cooked and shredded (3 ounces for men)

I piece string cheese, cut into rounds (1½ pieces for men)

½ ounce slivered almonds

Lettuce cups

Pile chicken, cheese, and almonds on top of lettuce cups. Eat cold.

Women: 235 cals; 15g fat; 6g carb; 23g protein
Men: 354 cals; 19g fat; 9g carb; 39g protein

Quinoa Bites with Zucchini, Tomato, and Arugula

Low-Carb Meal

2 tablespoons extra-virgin olive oil
2 tablespoons diced red onion
½ teaspoon minced garlic
½ medium zucchini, small dice
¼ teaspoon dried thyme
¼ teaspoon dried basil

¼ teaspoon ground black pepper
½ cup diced tomatoes
¾ cup cooked quinoa
1 handful of arugula, rinsed
6 whole eggs
6 egg whites

Heat olive oil over medium-high heat in a nonstick skillet.

Once oil is hot add onions, garlic, and zucchini. Add thyme, basil, and black pepper. Sauté until the vegetables are soft and have a light brown color. Add diced tomatoes, cooked quinoa, and arugula. Cook until arugula is wilted. Set aside and allow to cool.

Meanwhile, whisk together egg whites and whole eggs.

Generously spray muffin pan with cooking spray to prevent sticking. Preheat oven to 400 degrees.

Distribute 1½ tablespoons of vegetable mixture into each muffin cup.

Add egg mixture so that each cup is ¾ full.

Bake in preheated oven for approximately 20 minutes or until tops are light brown and the eggs are cooked through.

Makes 12 muffins

Women (3 muffins): 234 cals; 15g fat; 5g carb; 15g protein
Men (5 muffins): 390 cals; 25g fat; 8g carb; 25g protein

Salmon with Pesto "Zoodles"

Low-Carb Meal

I large zucchini squash

4 ounces wild caught salmon (6 ounces for men)

2 spears asparagus, chopped (4 spears for men)

I tablespoon pesto sauce (1½ tablespoons for men)

Lemon juice

Spiral slice or julienne-cut the zucchini to make "zoodles." Place in a strainer and liberally salt the zucchini; let sit 20 minutes (this helps your zucchini "sweat" out all its water).

Spray a frying pan with cooking spray and heat over medium heat.

Place the thawed salmon fillet on the pan. Cook for 5 minutes on each side or until salmon begins to flake. Remove from pan and set aside.

Thoroughly rinse salt off of the zucchini and pat dry. Spray another pan with cooking spray and cook "zoodles" and asparagus over medium heat until tender. Add pesto sauce to "zoodles" and top with salmon and a squirt of lemon juice. Enjoy!

Women: 270 cals; 16g fat; 8g carb; 25g protein
Men: 390 cals; 23g fat; 10g carb; 36g protein

Shrimp and Chicken Stir-Fry

Low-Carb Meal

I teaspoon coconut aminos

I tablespoon coconut oil

½ teaspoon minced garlic

½ cup shredded carrots

½ cup sugar snap pea pods, chopped

½ cup broccoli, chopped (1 cup for men)

½ cup mushrooms, sliced

6 cocktail shrimp, thawed (10 for men)

I ounce chicken breast, cubed (2 ounces for men)

I tablespoon green onions, sliced (2 tablespoons for men)

⅛ teaspoon black pepper

Heat the coconut aminos, coconut oil, and garlic in a skillet over medium-high heat. Add carrots once the oil is melted. Sauté for 5 minutes.

Add the remaining veggies, shrimp, and cubed chicken. Sauté an additional 10 minutes. Garnish with green onions and black pepper. Enjoy!

Women: 260 cals; 16g fat; 12g carb; 22g protein
Men: 360 cals; 17g fat; 17g carb; 39g protein

Shrimp Cocktail Salad

Low-Carb Meal

10 pieces large shrimp, halved
⅔ avocado, cubed (1 avocado for men)
1½ ounces chicken breast, cooked and cubed (for men only)

¼ cup cucumber, chopped
1 tablespoon cocktail sauce
1 tablespoon cilantro
Fresh lemon juice

Carefully mix shrimp, avocado, chicken (for men only), cucumber, cocktail sauce, cilantro, and lemon juice together in a small bowl. Eat cold.

Women: 240 cals; 15g fat; 13g carb; 17g protein
Men: 390 cals; 23g fat; 17g carb; 32g protein

Stuffed Avocado

Low-Carb Meal

½ medium-size avocado (¾ for men)
3 ounces cooked, shredded chicken (4 ounces for men)
2 tablespoons fat-free plain Greek yogurt

1 tablespoon Dijon mustard
Salt-free seasoning blend blend
Ground black pepper

Slice avocado in half and remove pit. Set aside.

Mix shredded chicken, yogurt, mustard, and seasonings together. Stuff mixture into the avocado. Eat with a spoon.

Women: 285 cals; 13g fat; 7g carb; 31g protein
Men: 390 cals; 20g fat; 10g carb; 40g protein

Taco Salad

Low-Carb Meal

Salad

2 ounces lean ground beef (4 ounces for men)

2 tablespoons yellow onion, chopped (¼ cup for men)

1 teaspoon homemade taco seasoning (2 teaspoons for men) (recipe below)

1½ cups romaine lettuce, chopped

½ cup chard, chopped

1 tablespoon olives, sliced

¼ avocado, sliced

1 tablespoon low-fat mozzarella cheese

1 tablespoon fat-free plain Greek yogurt

2 tablespoons fresh salsa

Chopped green onions

Heat skillet to medium-high heat.

Brown ground beef and onion together in skillet. Add taco seasoning.

To make salad, layer chopped romaine and chard, beef and onions, olives, avocado, cheese, Greek yogurt, salsa, and green onions. Enjoy!

Taco Seasoning

1 tablespoon chili powder

1 teaspoon cumin

½ teaspoon paprika

½ teaspoon black pepper

¼ teaspoon garlic powder

¼ teaspoon onion powder

¼ teaspoon crushed red pepper flakes

¼ teaspoon dried oregano

Mix all ingredients together and store in an airtight container. Remember to label it!

Women: 260 cals; 15g fat; 13g carb; 21g protein
Men: 390 cals; 21g fat; 14g carb; 36g protein

Thai-Style Turkey Cabbage Salad

Low-Carb Meal

Turkey

2 teaspoons coconut oil

3 ounces lean ground turkey (4 ounces for men)

1 teaspoon garlic, minced

1 tablespoon shallots, minced

¼ teaspoon salt substitute

¼ teaspoon black pepper

¼ teaspoon jalapeño, stems and seeds removed, minced

1 tablespoon rice vinegar, unseasoned

1 tablespoon lime juice

1 teaspoon Sriracha paste

In a nonstick skillet over high heat, melt the coconut oil and add turkey. Stir the turkey, making sure to break it up as you go.

Add the garlic, shallots, salt substitute, black pepper, jalapeños, vinegar, lime juice, and Sriracha paste.

Cook the turkey until it is cooked through all the way.

Cabbage

2 teaspoons extra-virgin olive oil

3 ounces yellow squash, ½-inch dice

3 ounces zucchini, ½-inch dice

Pinch of dried thyme

Pinch of red pepper flakes

Pinch of black pepper

In a skillet over high heat, heat olive oil. Add squash and zucchini and stir immediately. Keep stirring until vegetables have a light brown color and are fork tender. Add seasonings and remove from heat.

Women: 278 cals; 23g fat; 3g carb; 21g protein
Men: 344 cals; 26g fat; 3g carb; 28g protein

Vanilla Pecan Pudding

Low-Carb Meal

½ cup fat-free plain Greek yogurt (1 cup for men)

¼ cup vanilla protein powder

1 tablespoon all-natural almond butter

Vanilla stevia drops for sweetness

1 tablespoon chopped pecans (2 tablespoons for men)

Mix the Greek yogurt, protein powder, almond butter, and stevia together in a bowl. Top with pecans (or other nut of choice).

Women: 290 cals; 16g fat; 11g carb; 29g protein
Men: 410 cals; 21g fat; 16g carb; 41g protein

Vietnamese Grilled Chicken Spring Rolls with Sweet Ginger Lime Sauce

Low-Carb Meal

Spring Rolls

3 sheets rice paper wrapper

1 cup cabbage slaw

¼ avocado, sliced (½ avocado for men)

¼ cup shredded carrots

3 ounces grilled chicken, cut into long, thin strips (4 ounces for men)

¼ cucumber, shredded

3 green onions, just the cut-off white stem—leave whole

Basil and mint leaves (optional)

All ingredients will be divided between three rolls.

Run rice papers under hot water until they are flexible and soft.

With the rice paper flat on the cutting board, layer cabbage slaw, avocado, carrots, grilled chicken strips, shredded cucumber, and strip of green onion.

Roll the bottom of the sheet halfway up and cover ingredients.

Roll the left side toward the middle and do the same with the right side.

Ensuring paper is kept tight, roll tightly toward the top.
Repeat for the second and third roll. Top rolls with 1 serving of sauce (recipe follows).

Sauce

½ cup lime juice

1 teaspoon apple cider vinegar

¼ teaspoon Sriracha chili sauce

1½ tablespoons Truvia

½ teaspoon minced ginger

½ teaspoon minced garlic

Dash of salt substitute

¼ jalapeño, minced fine (optional)

Makes 2 servings

In a mixing bowl, whisk all ingredients together until Truvia is dissolved.

Women: 300 cals; 8g fat; 14g carb; 29g protein
Men: 400 cals; 15g fat; 17g carb; 38g protein

Zucchini and Turkey "Lasagna Roll-Ups"

Low-Carb Meal

Turkey Filling

1 tablespoon extra-virgin olive oil

1 tablespoon minced garlic

1 tablespoon yellow onion, minced

4 ounces lean ground turkey (5 ounces for men)

¼ teaspoon dried basil

¼ teaspoon dried oregano

¼ teaspoon dried thyme

¼ teaspoon black pepper

¼ teaspoon salt-free tomato basil seasoning

¼ teaspoon Truvia sweetener

½ cup diced canned tomatoes, no salt

In a nonstick skillet over medium heat, add the oil and sauté the garlic and onions until soft, stirring often. Add the ground turkey, basil, oregano, thyme, pepper, tomato basil seasoning, Truvia, and canned tomatoes. Simmer on medium until the turkey is cooked through. Set aside and allow to cool to room temperature.

Zucchini "Noodles"

1 medium zucchini, round and long   ¼ cup mozzarella cheese

Bring a large pot of water to boil.

Slice the zucchini lengthwise into ¼-inch strips.

Add the sliced zucchini to the boiling water and cook for about 4 minutes or until the zucchini strips are flexible without being mushy.

Remove them from the water and run under cold water until cool.

Lay the zucchini flat and divide the turkey mixture between 4 zucchini strips, placing mixture in the middle and rolling over until the end.

Place on a nonstick cookie sheet with a light spray of cooking spray.

Divide the cheese between the 4 roll-ups and broil on high until the cheese is melted and golden brown. Sprinkle with dried basil and serve.

Women: 280 cals; 16.5g fat; 4g carb; 34g protein
Men: 310 cals; 18g fat; 6g carb; 41g protein

CLEAN CHEAT MEALS

Banana Berry Ice Cream

Clean Cheat

1 cup 2% cottage cheese

½ cup berries (1 cup for men)

½ banana (1 banana for men)

2 tablespoons unsweetened almond milk

1 tablespoon nut butter

½ scoop vanilla protein powder

1 cup unsweetened almond milk

6 ice cubes (or 1 cup)

Natural sweetener of choice

The night before you intend to serve, blend cottage cheese, berries, banana, 2 tablespoons almond milk, nut butter, and protein powder. Pour into an ice cube tray and freeze overnight.

Place frozen cubes back in blender, and blend with 1 cup almond milk, ice cubes, and natural sweetener of choice, to desired sweetness. Enjoy!

Note: Make this the night before serving.

Women: 500 cals; 18g fat; 44g carb; 48g protein
Men: 607 cals; 19g fat; 70g carb; 49g protein

Barbecue Chicken Pita Pizza

Clean Cheat

1 whole-wheat flatbread
(1½ for men)

2 tablespoons reduced-sugar barbecue
sauce (3 tablespoons for men) (we like
the smoky mesquite flavor)

½ cup shredded Monterey jack and
cheddar cheese

2 ounces cooked and shredded chicken

Red onion, thinly sliced

Cilantro

Preheat oven to 350 degrees.

Spread the barbecue sauce on pita, then layer ¼ cup of cheese, chicken, red onion, cilantro, and remaining ¼ cup of cheese.

Bake on a baking sheet for 15–20 minutes. Enjoy!

Women: 495 cals; 16g fat; 53g carb; 40g protein
Men: 600 cals; 17g fat; 74g carb; 43g protein

BLT Burger and Sweet Potato Fries

Clean Cheat

½ cup sweet potatoes

Sea salt to taste

4 ounces beef

Dash each of salt, pepper, cumin, salt-free
seasoning blend, dried minced onion

1 slice nitrate-free turkey bacon

½ whole-grain bun (1 whole bun for men)

Lettuce

Tomato

1 tablespoon reduced-sugar barbecue
sauce

½ tablespoon olive oil mayo OR homemade mayo

Heat oven to 425 degrees. Heat grill or skillet to medium-high heat.

Slice ½ cup sweet potatoes into fries. Place a single layer of fries on a baking sheet lined with a crinkled and greased piece of tinfoil. Spray the tops with cooking spray or an olive oil misto and sprinkle with sea salt. Bake 15 minutes, flip. Bake another 15 minutes.

Mix beef and seasonings together with your hands and form a patty. Grill burger and bacon or cook on skillet to desired doneness.

Place burger patty on bun. Layer with bacon, lettuce, tomato, barbecue sauce, and mayo. (Women, leave off the top of the bun.) Eat fries on the side OR try to stack them on your burger. Enjoy!

Women: 496 cals; 22g fat; 41g carb; 31g protein
Men: 590 cals; 24g fat; 57g carb; 36g protein

Candied Pecan Protein Waffles

Clean Cheat

4 egg whites
¼ cup 2% cottage cheese
½ scoop vanilla protein powder
¼ banana (¾ banana for men)
⅓ cup oats (½ cup for men)

1 tablespoon ground flaxseed
1 teaspoon cinnamon
Topping:
1 tablespoon chopped pecans
2 tablespoons pure maple syrup

Heat waffle iron.

Blend egg whites, cottage cheese, protein powder, banana, oats, flaxseed, and cinnamon. Pour into a waffle iron that's been sprayed with cooking spray. Cook 2 minutes. Transfer to a plate.

Toast pecans in a frying pan over medium heat for 3–5 minutes. Add syrup to pan. Stir together. Once bubbles begin to form, pour over waffle. Enjoy!

Women: 525 cals; 13g fat; 66g carb; 41g protein
Men: 600 cals; 14g fat; 82g carb; 43g protein

Chocolate Glazed Crepes

Clean Cheat

Crepes

½ banana

½ cup oats (⅔ cup for men)

¼ cup unsweetened almond milk

1 whole egg

3 egg whites

1–2 teaspoons stevia

Dash of cinnamon

Chocolate Glaze

½ tablespoon almond butter

½ tablespoon coconut oil

1 tablespoon unsweetened almond milk

1 tablespoon raw honey

2 tablespoons chocolate protein powder

Topping (for men only):

½ banana, sliced

Spray a small frying pan with cooking spray and place over medium heat.

Blend the banana, oats, almond milk, eggs, stevia, and cinnamon for 2 minutes.

Pour ¼ of the batter into the frying pan and swirl around to cover base of the pan. Once bubbles form on the top, flip. Cook another minute, transfer to a plate and roll up. Should make 4 crepes.

For the glaze, place almond butter and coconut oil in a small bowl and heat for 20 seconds in the microwave. Stir in almond milk, honey, and protein powder. Drizzle over your crepes. Men, top with banana slices. Enjoy!

Women: 500 cals; 21g fat; 50g carb; 31g protein

Men: 603 cals; 22g fat; 72g carb; 33g protein

Chunky Monkey Bowl

Clean Cheat

¼ cup plain Greek yogurt
1 tablespoon peanut butter
1 frozen banana
½ scoop chocolate or vanilla protein
   powder (1 scoop for men)
4 ice cubes (or ½ cup)

Toppings:
½ banana, sliced
2 large strawberries, sliced
2 tablespoons granola
15 extra-dark chocolate chips
1 teaspoon raw honey

Blend yogurt, peanut butter, frozen banana, protein powder, and ice cubes.
Pour in a bowl and top with all toppings. Enjoy!

Women: 492 cals; 14g fat; 72g carb; 28g protein
Men: 562 cals; 15g fat; 74g carb; 41g protein

Homemade Oreos

Clean Cheat

Cookies

6 tablespoons whole-wheat flour
2 tablespoons chocolate protein powder
1 tablespoon cocoa powder
Dash of sea salt

2 tablespoons melted coconut oil
3 tablespoons pure maple syrup
1 whole egg
¼ teaspoon pure vanilla extract

Cream Filling

¼ cup full-fat whipped cream cheese
2 tablespoons vanilla protein powder

¼ teaspoon pure vanilla extract
½ tablespoon pure maple syrup

Preheat oven to 325 degrees. Line a baking sheet with parchment paper.

Sift together the flour, chocolate protein powder, cocoa powder, and salt. Set aside. Beat together the melted coconut oil and maple syrup. Add egg and vanilla. Mix. Add dry ingredients to wet ingredients. Mix.

Scoop into 1-inch balls and place on baking sheet; this should make 8 cookies. Bake for 7–9 minutes. Transfer to a cooling rack.

Beat together all ingredients for the cream filling. Once cookies are cooled, spoon 1 tablespoon filling onto each of 4 cookies and sandwich with the remaining 4 cookies. Enjoy!

Makes 4 cookies

Women (2 cookies): 445 cals; 24g fat; 49g carb; 16g protein
Men (3 cookies): 665 cals; 36g fat; 73g carb; 23g protein

Hootenanny Pancakes

Clean Cheat

Pancakes

½ tablespoon coconut oil

4 egg whites

1 whole egg

½ cup Kodiak Cakes pancake mix

½ cup unsweetened almond milk

¼ teaspoon sea salt

¼ teaspoon pure vanilla extract

Toppings:

¼ cup sliced strawberries (½ cup for men)

1 tablespoon heavy whipping cream (2 tablespoons for men)

½ tablespoon pure maple syrup (1 tablespoon for men)

Preheat oven to 425 degrees. Spray an 8 x 8-inch baking pan with cooking spray. Place the coconut oil in the pan and put in the oven to melt.

Place all the other ingredients except the toppings in a blender and blend for 5 minutes (do not skip this step!).

Pull the pan out of the oven and pour the blended mixture into the melted coconut oil.

Return the pan to oven and bake for 20 minutes. Top with strawberries, cream, and syrup. Enjoy!!

Women: 492 cals; 21g fat; 41g carb; 35g protein
Men: 599 cals; 27g fat; 55g carb; 36g protein

Mac and Cheese with Bacon

Clean Cheat

3 ounces brown rice pasta (4 ounces for men)

2 tablespoons minced onion

½ teaspoon minced garlic

Dash of cayenne pepper

¼ cup reserved pasta water

⅓ cup 2% cheddar cheese

2 tablespoons plain Greek yogurt

1 slice turkey bacon, chopped

1 tablespoon whole-grain breadcrumbs

1 tablespoon Parmesan cheese

Preheat oven to 425 degrees. Cook the pasta a couple minutes using the package directions. Add a pinch of sea salt to the water. Once cooked, drain and save ¼ cup of the pasta water.

Sauté the onions, garlic, and cayenne pepper in a small frying pan over medium-high heat. Once the onions are soft, add ¼ cup of your pasta water to the pan and lower heat to low-medium. Then add the cheddar cheese and stir until melted. Turn to low heat.

Return pasta to its original pot without any heat. Add yogurt, bacon, melted cheese mixture from the frying pan, and salt and pepper to taste. Mix well.

Pour into a small baking dish. Top with breadcrumbs and Parmesan cheese. Bake for 10 minutes or until cheese is melted. Enjoy!!

Women: 505 cals; 17g fat; 69g carb; 25g protein
Men: 602 cals; 19g fat; 90g carb; 27g protein

Muddy Buddies

Clean Cheat

1½ tablespoons peanut butter (2 tablespoons for men)

3 tablespoons honey

½ teaspoon cocoa powder

2 tablespoons chocolate protein powder

1 cup corn or rice Chex cereal (1½ cups for men)

2 tablespoons peanut butter powder

Melt peanut butter and honey together in the microwave for 20 seconds in a medium-size bowl. Stir in cocoa powder and protein powder. Add Chex and coat well.

Pour mixture into a zip-lock bag. Add peanut butter powder, seal bag, and shake until well coated. Enjoy!

Women: 500 cals; 14g fat; 89g carb; 21g protein
Men: 597 cals; 18g fat; 103g carb; 24g protein

One-Minute Brownie

Clean Cheat

1 whole egg	¼ teaspoon sea salt
1 tablespoon pure maple syrup	¼ teaspoon baking powder
1 tablespoon unsweetened almond milk	10 extra-dark chocolate chips (20 chips for men)
2 tablespoons nut butter	2 tablespoons heavy cream sweetened with stevia (3 tablespoons for men)
½ scoop chocolate protein powder	
1 tablespoon cocoa powder	

Beat together the egg, maple syrup, almond milk, and nut butter. Add the protein powder, cocoa powder, sea salt, baking powder, and chocolate chips. Mix well.

Pour into a microwave-safe bowl that's been sprayed with cooking spray and microwave for 1 minute. Top with cream and enjoy!

Women: 538 cals; 36g fat; 33g carb; 25g protein
Men: 615 cals; 43g fat; 36g carb; 26g protein

Peanut Butter Chocolate Chip Cookie Dough

Clean Cheat

2 tablespoons peanut butter (2½ tablespoons for men)	2 tablespoons vanilla protein powder
1 tablespoon raw honey (2 tablespoons for men)	⅓ cup oat flour
¼ teaspoon pure vanilla extract	15 extra-dark chocolate chips

Mix all ingredients together and eat as is OR scoop into cookie dough balls. Enjoy!

Women: 495 cals; 33g fat; 34g carb; 20g protein
Men: 599 cals; 26g fat; 73g carb; 23g protein

Pigs in a Blanket

Clean Cheat

½ cup Kodiak Cakes pancake mix (¾ cup for men)

½ tablespoon olive oil (1 tablespoon for men)

2 tablespoons warm water (3 tablespoons for men)

1 large chicken sausage

2 tablespoons ketchup

Side salad (optional)

Preheat oven to 450 degrees. Line a baking sheet with parchment paper.

Mix together Kodiak Cakes mix, olive oil, and warm water until the mixture resembles bread dough.

Wrap dough around the chicken sausage. Place on a baking sheet and bake for 10 minutes. Dip in ketchup. Enjoy a side salad with your meal.

Women: 430 cals; 17g fat; 40g carb; 30g protein
Men: 585 cals; 25g fat; 55g carb; 37g protein

Spinach Artichoke Dip with Pita Chips

Clean Cheat

1 cup spinach, finely chopped

5 ounces canned artichoke hearts, chopped

⅓ cup Parmesan cheese

⅓ cup mozzarella cheese

⅔ cup plain Greek yogurt

½ teaspoon minced garlic

½ teaspoon lemon juice

½ teaspoon salt-free seasoning blend

12 Stacy's pita chips (20 chips for men)

Preheat oven to 375 degrees.

Mix the spinach, artichokes, Parmesan, and mozzarella in a medium-size bowl. In a separate bowl, mix the yogurt, garlic, lemon juice, and seasonings. Add the yogurt mixture to the cheese and spinach mixture. Mix well.

Pour into a greased 8 x 8-inch baking pan that's been sprayed with cooking spray. Bake for 25 minutes or until the cheese is golden around the edges.

Sprinkle the top with Parmesan cheese when finished and enjoy with pita chips!

Women: 511 cals; 21g fat; 35g carb; 41g protein
Men: 615 cals; 25g fat; 51g carb; 43g protein

Sweet Potato Nachos

Clean Cheat

6 ounces sweet potatoes, very thinly
  sliced (10 ounces for men)
⅓ cup Monterey jack and cheddar cheese
4 ounces lean ground turkey, cooked
1 teaspoon taco seasoning
1 tablespoon guacamole

1 tablespoon salsa
1 tablespoon plain Greek yogurt
2 tablespoons sliced olives
Jalapeño slices (optional)
Green onions (optional)

Preheat oven to 250 degrees. Line a baking sheet with parchment paper. Place the sweet potato slices in a single layer on the baking sheet. Bake for 1 hour. If they are still soft, flip and bake an additional 15 minutes.

Transfer hot sweet potato chips to a plate and top with cheese, hot ground turkey, taco seasoning, guacamole, salsa, yogurt, olives, jalapeños, and green onions. Dig in!

Women: 500 cals; 22g fat; 42g carb; 34g protein
Men: 600 cals; 23g fat; 66g carb; 36g protein

Appendices

APPENDIX A
21-Day Daily Tracker

⬆ DAY 1
(HIGH CARB)

MEALS
Note what went well, struggles, likes, and dislikes.

☐
☐
☐
☐
☐

FITNESS TEST
Do each exercise for 1 min. Record # done.
Push-ups:
Sit-ups:
Squats:
Burpees:

GO THE DISTANCE
What round did you get to?

MIGHTY MINUTES
5-minute *minimum* then record progress.

LESSON INSIGHTS
Find Your *What* and Your *Why*
Record your thoughts and insights below.

⬆ DAY 2
(HIGH CARB)

MEALS
Note what went well, struggles, likes, and dislikes.

☐
☐
☐
☐
☐

THE WHOLE 9
What was your time?

DIRTY TWO-THIRTIES
5-minute *minimum* then record progress.

LESSON INSIGHTS
Discover the True Path to Transformation
Record your thoughts and insights below.

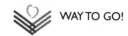 WAY TO GO!

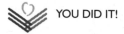 YOU DID IT!

EXTREME TRANSFORMATION • 21-DAY TRACKER

⬆ DAY 3
HIGH CARB

MEALS //
Note what went well, struggles, likes, and dislikes.

⬜
⬜
⬜
⬜
⬜

BURPEE LOVE ////////////////////////////////
What was your time?

MISSION

THRILLING THIRTIES ///////////////////////
5-minute *minimum* then record progress.

ACCELERATOR

LESSON INSIGHTS ///////////////////////////
Keep Your Promises
Record your thoughts and insights below.

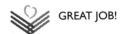 GREAT JOB!

⬆ DAY 4
HIGH CARB

MEALS //
Note what went well, struggles, likes, and dislikes.

⬜
⬜
⬜
⬜
⬜

PHOENIX RISING ////////////////////////////
How many rounds did you get?

MISSION

TENACIOUS TWOS ///////////////////////////
5-minute *minimum* then record progress.

ACCELERATOR

LESSON INSIGHTS ///////////////////////////
Prepare for Success
Record your thoughts and insights below.

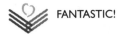 FANTASTIC!

EXTREME TRANSFORMATION • 21-DAY TRACKER

⬇ DAY 5

MEALS ////////////////////////////////////
Note what went well, struggles, likes, and dislikes.

☐
☐
☐
☐
☐

A LOTTA TABATA ////////////////////////
What was your lowest rep count per round for each exercise?

NASTY NINETIES ////////////////////////
5-minute *minimum* then record progress.

LESSON INSIGHTS ////////////////////////
Rally Your Team
Record your thoughts and insights below.

⬇ DAY 6

MEALS ////////////////////////////////////
Note what went well, struggles, likes, and dislikes.

☐
☐
☐
☐
☐

MIGHTY MINUTES ////////////////////////
5-minute *minimum* then record progress.

LESSON INSIGHTS ////////////////////////
Make It Your Own!
Record your thoughts and insights below.

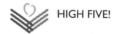 HIGH FIVE!

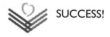 SUCCESS!

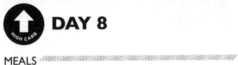

EXTREME TRANSFORMATION • 21-DAY TRACKER

 DAY 7

 DAY 8

MEALS
Note what went well, struggles, likes, and dislikes.

MEALS
Note what went well, struggles, likes, and dislikes.

 WEIGH IN
Start your day by weighing in and
record your weight. How did you do?

 THE GRINDER
What was your time?

 LESSON INSIGHTS
Troubleshoot!
Record your thoughts and insights below.

 DIRTY TWO-THIRTIES
10-minute *minimum* then record progress.

LESSON INSIGHTS
Believe In Yourself
Record your thoughts and insights below.

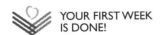 YOUR FIRST WEEK
IS DONE!

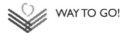 WAY TO GO!

EXTREME TRANSFORMATION • 21-DAY TRACKER

⬆ DAY 9

MEALS
Note what went well, struggles, likes, and dislikes.

☐
☐
☐
☐
☐

RUNNIN' WILD
What was your time?

THRILLING THIRTIES
10-minute *minimum* then record progress.

LESSON INSIGHTS
Be Open, Honest, and Vulnerable
Record your thoughts and insights below.

⬆ DAY 10

MEALS
Note what went well, struggles, likes, and dislikes.

☐
☐
☐
☐
☐

MT. EVEREST
What was your time?

TENACIOUS TWOS
10-minute *minimum* then record progress.

LESSON INSIGHTS
Unload the Real Weight
Record your thoughts and insights below.

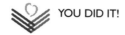 YOU DID IT!

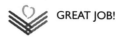 GREAT JOB!

EXTREME TRANSFORMATION • 21-DAY TRACKER

⬆ DAY 11
HIGH CARB

MEALS
Note what went well, struggles, likes, and dislikes.

☐
☐
☐
☐
☐

HUSTLE TIME
MISSION
How many rounds did you get?

NASTY NINETIES
ACCELERATOR
10-minute *minimum* then record progress.

LESSON INSIGHTS
Banish the Negative Self-Talk
Record your thoughts and insights below.

⬇ DAY 12
LOW CARB

MEALS
Note what went well, struggles, likes, and dislikes.

☐
☐
☐
☐
☐

BREAKTHROUGH
MISSION
What was your lowest rep count per round for each exercise?

MIGHTY MINUTES
ACCELERATOR
10-minute *minimum* then record progress.

LESSON INSIGHTS
Create Your New Identity
Record your thoughts and insights below.

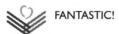 FANTASTIC!

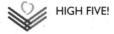 HIGH FIVE!

EXTREME TRANSFORMATION • 21-DAY TRACKER

 DAY 13

MEALS ///
Note what went well, struggles, likes, and dislikes.

☐
☐
☐
☐
☐

DIRTY TWO-THIRTIES ///////////////////////////
10-minute *minimum* then record progress.

LESSON INSIGHTS ///////////////////////////
Take Responsibility
Record your thoughts and insights below.

 DAY 14

MEALS ///
Note what went well, struggles, likes, and dislikes.

☐
☐
☐
☐
☐

WEIGH IN ///////////////////////////////////
Start your day by weighing in and
record your weight. How did you do?

LESSON INSIGHTS ///////////////////////////
Conquer Your F.E.AR.
Record your thoughts and insights below.

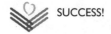 SUCCESS!

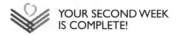 YOUR SECOND WEEK
IS COMPLETE!

EXTREME TRANSFORMATION • 21-DAY TRACKER

⬆ DAY 15

MEALS
Note what went well, struggles, likes, and dislikes.

☐
☐
☐
☐
☐

THE COUNTDOWN
What was your time?

THRILLING THIRTIES
15-minute *minimum* then record progress.

LESSON INSIGHTS
Go All In
Record your thoughts and insights below.

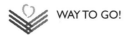 WAY TO GO!

⬆ DAY 16

MEALS
Note what went well, struggles, likes, and dislikes.

☐
☐
☐
☐
☐

AFTERBURNER
What was your time?

TENACIOUS TWOS
15-minute *minimum* then record progress.

LESSON INSIGHTS
Fall Without Failing
Record your thoughts and insights below.

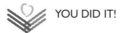 YOU DID IT!

EXTREME TRANSFORMATION • 21-DAY TRACKER

⬆ DAY 17
HIGH CARB

MEALS
Note what went well, struggles, likes, and dislikes.

☐
☐
☐
☐
☐

CHIPPIN' AWAY
MISSION
What was your time?

NASTY NINETIES
ACCELERATOR
15-minute *minimum* then record progress.

LESSON INSIGHTS
Be Beneficially Selfish
Record your thoughts and insights below.

⬆ DAY 18
HIGH CARB

MEALS
Note what went well, struggles, likes, and dislikes.

☐
☐
☐
☐
☐

GO TIME
MISSION
How many rounds did you get?

MIGHTY MINUTES
ACCELERATOR
15-minute *minimum* then record progress.

LESSON INSIGHTS
Have Realistic Expectations of Others
Record your thoughts and insights below.

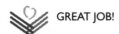 GREAT JOB!

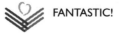 FANTASTIC!

EXTREME TRANSFORMATION • 21-DAY TRACKER

 DAY 19

MEALS
Note what went well, struggles, likes, and dislikes.

 WAKE-UP CALL
What was your lowest rep count per round for each exercise?

DIRTY TWO-THIRTIES
15-minute *minimum* then record progress.

LESSON INSIGHTS
Replace Your Addiction
Record your thoughts and insights below.

 DAY 20

MEALS
Note what went well, struggles, likes, and dislikes.

THRILLING THIRTIES
15-minute *minimum* then record progress.

LESSON INSIGHTS
Triggers and Tactics
Record your thoughts and insights below.

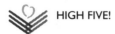 HIGH FIVE!

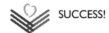 SUCCESS!

EXTREME TRANSFORMATION • 21-DAY TRACKER

DAY 21

MEALS

Note what went well, struggles, likes, and dislikes.

- [ ]
- [ ]
- [ ]
- [ ]
- [ ]

WEIGH IN

Start your day by weighing in and record your weight. How did you do?

LESSON INSIGHTS

Live with Purpose

Record your thoughts and insights below.

PHASE 2

DAYS 22–42

Repeat Days 1-21 following the same meals and missions and reviewing each daily lesson.

INCREASE TIMES

Repeat each day's accelerator workout but increase the number of minutes each week.

DAYS 1–6	20 minutes
DAYS 8–13	25 minutes
DAYS 15–20	30 minutes

PHASE 3

DAYS 43–63

Repeat Days 1-21 following the same meals and missions and reviewing each daily lesson.

INCREASE TIMES

Repeat each day's accelerator workout but increase the number of minutes each week.

DAYS 1–6	35 minutes
DAYS 8–13	40 minutes
DAYS 15–20	45 minutes

PHASE 4

DAYS 64–84

Repeat Days 1-21 following the same meals and missions and reviewing each daily lesson.

INCREASE TIMES

Repeat each day's accelerator workout but increase the number of minutes each week.

DAYS 1–6	50 minutes
DAYS 8–13	55 minutes
DAYS 15–20	60 minutes

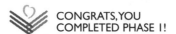

CONGRATS, YOU COMPLETED PHASE 1!

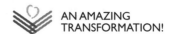

AN AMAZING TRANSFORMATION!

APPENDIX B
Shopping Lists and Meal Prep

We've created these Shopping Lists, separated by women and men, to give you an organized week-by-week list of what foods you'll need during your Extreme Transformation, including lists for Clean Cheat days. There's a separate Meal Prep Guide as well, so that after you bring home all the delicious ingredients, you can eliminate the guesswork by planning and prepping your meals ahead of time.

Shopping Lists

Week 1 Shopping List

PROTEIN

Women	Men	Item	Women	Men	Item	Women	Men	Item
8	12	whole eggs	7	11	scoops protein powder	6	8	ounces organic lean ground beef
8	10	egg whites	22	35	ounces chicken breasts	4	6	ounces white fish
12	16	ounces low-sodium cottage cheese	12	13	ounces extra-lean ground turkey	3	5	ounces wild caught salmon
10	40	ounces fat-free plain Greek yogurt	4	4	ounces nitrate-free turkey bacon	6	10	large shrimp

FRUIT

Women	Men	Item	Women	Men	Item	Women	Men	Item
6	7	bananas	1	1	apple	6	8	ounces blackberries
3	1	lemons	6	14	ounces strawberries	4	6	ounces blueberries
5	5	limes	8	10	ounces raspberries			

VEGGIES AND HERBS

Women	Men	Item	Women	Men	Item	Women	Men	Item
20	20	ounces fresh green beans	1	1	yellow beet	1	1	bunch parsley
4	4	ounces shredded carrots	1	1	large yellow onion	1	1	bunch chives
1	1	package alfalfa sprouts	1	1	large red onion	2	2	bunches green onions
1	1	cup shredded kale	1	1	green bell pepper	1	1	bunch cilantro
4	5	cups spinach	2	2	red bell peppers	1	1	bunch fresh basil (optional)
1	1	5-ounce can artichoke hearts	4	4	ounces sugar snap peas	1	1	bunch fresh mint (optional)
1	1	romaine lettuce heart	8	12	ounces mushrooms	1	1	small bag frozen corn
1	1	head chard	1	1	zucchini	1	1	small jar minced garlic
1	1	head butter lettuce	2	2	cucumbers	10	10	ounces fresh salsa
3	4	cups cabbage slaw	1	1	bunch asparagus spears	1	1	16-ounce can diced tomatoes, no salt
2	2	celery stalks	1	1	tomato	1	1	6-ounce can tomato paste
1	1	head cauliflower	8	8	ounces edamame			
1	1	head broccoli	1	1	jalapeño			

CARBOHYDRATES

Women	Men	Item	Women	Men	Item	Women	Men	Item
1	1	loaf Ezekiel low-sodium bread (frozen section)	3	4	sweet potatoes	1	2	Ezekiel tortilla(s)
½	½	cup Kodiak Cakes pancake mix	4	5	small red potatoes			Kashi GoLean Crisp cereal
1	1	whole-grain bun	16	16	ounces butternut squash			rice paper wrapper
1	1	15-ounce can garbanzo beans, no salt	16	20	ounces old-fashioned rolled oats			Stacy's pita chips
1	2	15-ounce can(s) black beans, no salt	1	1	small bag brown rice			extra-dark chocolate chips
			3	4	yellow corn tortillas			granola (optional)

FAT

Women	Men	Item	Women	Men	Item	Women	Men	Item
		heavy whipping cream	1	1	6-ounce container Laughing Cow cheese wedges	3	4	tablespoons all-natural peanut butter
		extra-virgin olive oil	½	½	slice low-sodium cheddar	1	1	serving(s) all-natural almond butter (see product label)
		coconut oil	2½	2½	ounces Parmesan cheese			almond flour
		low-fat mayonnaise	2	2	ounces sliced or slivered almonds			milled flaxseed
1	1	2¼-ounce can sliced olives	1	2	ounce(s) chopped pecans	0	1	ounce chopped hazelnuts
3	4	avocados						
10½	10½	ounces low-fat mozzarella cheese						

SEASONINGS

salt-free seasoning blend	smoked paprika	poppy seeds
salt-free tomato & garlic seasoning	ground ginger	ground mustard
salt-free garlic & herb seasoning	garlic powder	nutmeg
salt-free tomato basil seasoning	dried minced onion	cinnamon
salt-free onion & herb seasoning	onion powder	dried basil
salt substitute	crushed red pepper flakes	dried oregano
ground black pepper	dried basil	dried thyme
ground cumin	chili powder	sea salt

MISCELLANEOUS ITEMS

Women	Men	Item	Item	Item
24	28	ounces unsweetened almond milk	Sriracha chili sauce	baking soda
8	8	ounces low-sodium chicken broth	Dijon mustard	pure vanilla extract
8	8	ounces unsweetened applesauce	reduced-sugar barbecue sauce	almond extract (optional)
		raw honey	peanut butter powder	Truvia
		sugar-free syrup	apple cider vinegar	vanilla liquid stevia drops
		pure maple syrup	coconut aminos	

EXTREME TRANSFORMATION MEAL PREP—WEEK I

Days 1–3

Cook 12 ounces boneless, skinless chicken breast (20 ounces for men)

Cook 4 ounces extra-lean ground turkey

Cook ¼ cup brown rice (⅓ cup for men)

Make Lemon Poppy Seed Protein Bites (freeze extras)

Make Tomato Salsa

Thaw shrimp in fridge (see recipe for amount)

Days 4–6

Cook 10 ounces boneless, skinless chicken breast (15 ounces for men)

Cook 4 ounces extra-lean ground turkey (5 ounces for men)

Cook 2 ounces lean ground beef (4 ounces for men)

Bake 5 ounces sweet potatoes, cut into 4 rounds (6 ounces for men)

Bake ½ cup sweet potatoes, whole (¾ cup for men)

Make Taco Seasoning

Make Sweet Ginger Lime Sauce

Place salmon in fridge to thaw (see recipe for amount)

Marinate 4 ounces white fish in fridge for Citrus and Onion Fish Tacos

Week 2 Shopping List

Go through your cupboards and cross off anything that you may already have.

PROTEIN

Women	Men	Item	Women	Men	Item	Women	Men	Item
7	8	whole eggs	3	6½	scoops protein powder	1	2	ounce(s) organic lean ground beef
15	21	egg whites	13	22½	ounces chicken breast	12	17	ounces wild caught salmon
33	37	ounces fat-free plain Greek yogurt	9	12	ounces extra-lean ground turkey	4	6	ounces wild tuna
6	10	ounces low-sodium, fat-free cottage cheese	1–2	1–2	slices nitrate-free turkey bacon	4	5	ounces tilapia

FRUITS

Women	Men	Item	Women	Men	Item	Women	Men	Item
1	1	pineapple	1	2	large orange(s)	12	16	ounces blackberries
3	3	limes	5	6	bananas	4	8	ounces raspberries
4	4	lemons	12	24	ounces blueberries	1	1	apple

VEGGIES AND HERBS

Women	Men	Item	Women	Men	Item	Women	Men	Item
8	8	ounces fresh green beans	1	1	green bell pepper	1	1	bunch fresh basil
1	2	head(s) cauliflower	2	2	bunches asparagus spears	1	1	bunch fresh parsley
1	1	head broccoli	12	16	ounces sugar snap peas	1	1	bunch cilantro
1	1	head green cabbage	1	1	cucumber	4	4	small mint leaves
1	1	head red cabbage	1	1	spaghetti squash	1	1	bunch green onions
4	4	cups spinach	2	2	cherry tomatoes	1	1	bunch chives
1	1	yellow onion	6	6	ounces raw edamame, shelled			fresh ginger
2	2	red onions	2	2	medium poblano peppers	1	1	shallot
4	4	ounces frozen corn	1	1	jalapeño			minced garlic
2	2	zucchini	1	1	small green tomatillo	4	4	ounces fresh salsa
1	1	yellow squash	6	6	sprigs fresh tarragon			
2	2	red bell peppers	1	1	sprig rosemary			

CARBOHYDRATES

Women	Men	Item	Women	Men	Item	Women	Men	Item
7	10	ounces sweet potatoes	4	4	slices Ezekiel low-sodium bread (frozen section)	2	3	rice cakes
3	4	small red potatoes	1	1	whole-wheat pita (Papa Pita brand)			Kashi GoLean Crisp cereal
6	9	ounces quinoa			whole-grain bread crumbs			Corn Chex cereal
6	12	ounces brown rice	3	3	ounces whole-wheat flour	11	12	ounces old-fashioned rolled oats
3	3	ounces brown rice pasta	3	3	yellow corn tortillas			dark chocolate chips
1	1	15-ounce can black beans						

FATS

Women	Men	Item	Women	Men	Item	Women	Men	Item
2	2	ounces whipped cream cheese	4	4	ounces cheddar jack cheese	1	1	ounce pistachios
1	1	ounce reduced-fat unsweetened shredded coconut	2	2	slices pepper jack cheese	2	2	ounces raw pumpkin seeds
4	4	ounces low-fat mozzarella cheese			low-fat mayonnaise	1	1	2¼-ounce can sliced olives
1	1	ounce shredded Parmesan cheese			pesto sauce			all-natural almond butter
2	2	tablespoons feta cheese			coconut oil			all-natural peanut butter
6	6	ounces cheddar cheese			extra-virgin olive oil	1	1½	tablespoon unsalted butter
			5	5	ounces slivered almonds			milled flaxseed

SEASONINGS

sea salt	dried thyme	dried oregano
black pepper	red pepper flakes	cayenne pepper
salt-free garlic & herb seasoning	cocoa powder	granulated garlic
salt-free southwest seasoning	powdered peanut butter	garlic powder
salt-free tomato basil seasoning	cinnamon	ground mustard
salt-free chicken seasoning	nutmeg	onion powder
salt-free onion & herb seasoning	paprika	dried minced onion
salt substitute	cumin	

MISCELLANEOUS ITEMS

Women	Men	Item	Women	Men	Item	Women	Men	Item
		raw honey			rice vinegar	8	8	ounces unsweetened applesauce
		pure maple syrup			Sriracha chili sauce			Dijon mustard
		vanilla liquid stevia drops	36	36	ounces unsweetened almond milk			reduced-sugar barbecue sauce
		pure vanilla extract			powdered peanut butter			apple cider vinegar
		coconut extract (optional)			zero-calorie nonstick cooking spray			
		Truvia						

EXTREME TRANSFORMATION MEAL PREP—WEEK 2

Days 8–10

Cook 1 ounce lean ground beef (2 ounces for men)

Cook 2 ounces boneless, skinless chicken breast (3 ounces for men)

Cook 6 ounces extra-lean ground turkey (8 ounces for men)

Cook ¼ cup quinoa (½ cup for men)

Cook ¾ cup brown rice (1½ cups for men)

Boil 4 eggs (6 eggs for men)

Make Pumpkin Seed Granola (refrigerate extras)

Make Berry Puree

Thaw salmon in fridge (see recipe for amount)

Thaw and marinate tuna in fridge (see recipe for amount)

Days 11–13

Cook 6 ounces boneless, skinless chicken breast (12 ounces for men)

Cook 1 cup quinoa

Bake ½ cup sweet potatoes, whole (¾ cup for men)

Boil 1 cup red potatoes (1½ cups for men)

Boil 7 eggs (10 eggs for men)

Make Marinade for chicken

Make Yogurt Sauce

Make Greek Yogurt Tartar Sauce

Make Chocolate Chip Almond Coconut Bites (freeze extras)

Make Hummus

Thaw 3 ounces extra-lean ground turkey in fridge (4 ounces for men)

Week 3 Shopping List

Go through your cupboards and cross off anything that you may already have.

PROTEIN

Women	Men	Item	Women	Men	Item	Women	Men	Item
13	13	whole eggs	26	34	ounces fat-free plain Greek yogurt	3	5	ounces lean lamb meat (shoulder)
18	20	egg whites	1	1	large chicken sausage	2	4	pieces firm tofu
6½	11	scoops protein powder	6½	16½	ounces chicken breast	2	4	ounces canned tuna
10	10	ounces cottage cheese	14	22	ounces extra-lean ground turkey	3	5	ounces wild caught salmon
		protein powder	3	5	ounces lean pork tenderloin	10	10	large shrimp

FRUITS

Women	Men	Item	Women	Men	Item	Women	Men	Item
3	3	limes	1	1	pear	20	20	ounces strawberries
2	2	lemons	8	10	bananas	12	12	ounces blackberries
2	2	apples	1	2	large orange(s)	4	4	ounces berries of choice

VEGGIES AND HERBS

Women	Men	Item	Women	Men	Item	Women	Men	Item
4	4	tomatoes on the vine	2	2	yellow onions	2	2	ounces pumpkin puree
1	1	head broccoli	2	2	red onions			minced garlic
1	1	head cauliflower	4	4	red bell peppers			fresh salsa
1	1	cup cabbage or cabbage slaw	1	1	green bell pepper			fresh rosemary
1	1	romaine lettuce heart	1	1	jalapeño (optional)	1	1	bunch cilantro
		Boston, Bibb, or red leaf lettuce	1	1	bunch asparagus spears	1	1	bunch parsley
2	2	cups arugula	8	8	ounces fresh green beans	4	4	small mint leaves
4	4	cups spinach	1	1	radish	1	1	basil leaf
1	1	eggplant	2	2	small mushrooms	3	3	small sage leaves
2	2	cucumbers	10	10	cherry tomatoes	1	1	bunch green onions
3	3	zucchini squash	2	2	ounces edamame, shelled	1	1	bunch chives
2	2	yellow squash	2	2	ounces frozen or fresh corn	3	3	sprigs tarragon

CARBOHYDRATES

Women	Men	Item	Women	Men	Item	Women	Men	Item
8	8	ounces whole-wheat flour			Kodiak Cakes pancake mix	6	6	ounces old-fashioned rolled oats
14	14	ounces quinoa, cooked	1	1	spelt tortilla (Rudi's brand)	2	3	rice cakes
16	22	ounces sweet potatoes	2	2	ounces black beans			extra-dark chocolate chips
1	1	small sweet potato	6	8	ounces white beans			
6	8	ounces red potatoes	2	2	ounces steel-cut oats			

FAT

Women	Men	Item	Women	Men	Item	Women	Men	Item
		heavy whipping cream	1	2	piece(s) string cheese	3	4	ounces milled flaxseed or chia seeds
		coconut oil	2	2	ounces raw peanuts, unsalted			all-natural nut butter of choice
6	6	ounces low-fat mozzarella cheese	1	1	ounce chopped pecans			
4	4	ounces fat-free cheddar cheese	4	5	avocados	1	1	ounce sliced olives
3	3	ounces cheddar jack cheese			extra-virgin olive oil			
			1½	2½	ounces slivered almonds			

SEASONINGS

cinnamon	granulated garlic	red pepper flakes
sea salt	cumin seed	ground cumin
salt substitute	yellow mustard seed	onion powder
salt-free garlic & herb seasoning	ground mustard powder	dried oregano
salt-free tomato basil seasoning	ground turmeric	dried basil
salt-free onion & herb seasoning	ground ginger	whole fennel seeds
salt-free southwest seasoning	yellow curry powder	dried thyme
salt-free chicken seasoning	ground coriander	ground nutmeg
paprika	garam masala	ketchup
black pepper	chili powder	
garlic powder	red chili flakes	

MISCELLANEOUS ITEMS

Women	Men	Item	Women	Men	Item	Women	Men	Item
		zero-calorie nonstick cooking spray			powdered peanut butter	8	8	ounces unsweetened applesauce
8	8	ounces black coffee			vanilla liquid stevia drops			cocktail sauce
		Dijon mustard			reduced-sugar barbecue sauce	8	8	ounces low-sodium chicken broth
		pure vanilla extract	22	22	ounces unsweetened almond milk			cocoa powder
		Truvia baking powder			balsamic vinegar			
					sugar-free pancake syrup			

EXTREME TRANSFORMATION MEAL PREP—WEEK 3

Days 15–17

Cook 4 ounces extra-lean ground turkey (5 ounces for men)

Cook 1 ounce boneless, skinless chicken breast (3 ounces for men)

Bake 6 ounces sweet potatoes, 4 rounds (8 ounces for men)

Bake ½ cup sweet potatoes, diced (¾ cup for men)

Make Strawberry and Banana Quinoa Muffins (freeze extras)

Make Cilantro Lime Dressing

Thaw 3 ounces pork on Day 16 (5 ounces for men) (marinate in refrigerator overnight)

Thaw 7 ounces extra-lean ground turkey in fridge (10 ounces for men)

Days 18–20

Cook 1½ ounces boneless, skinless chicken breast (3 ounces for men)

Cook 2 ounces extra-lean ground turkey (4 ounces for men)

Cook ¾ cup quinoa

Bake 6 ounces red potatoes (8 ounces for men)

Make Homemade Ranch Powder

Make Berry Puree

Make Avocado Puree

Make House Pickles

Make Breakfast Frittata Veggie "Muffins"

Marinate 3 ounces lamb in All-Purpose Marinade in fridge (5 ounces for men)

Thaw 3 ounces extra-lean ground turkey in fridge (5 ounces for men)

APPENDIX C
Extreme Transformation Bulk Prep Cooking Guide

Bulk Prep Cooking Guide

PROTEIN

Chicken

Grill

1. Preheat outdoor or countertop grill on high heat.
2. Lightly spray the grill with nonstick cooking spray.
3. Grill 12–15 minutes per side.
4. Chicken is done when it is no longer pink and juices run clear.
5. Add seasonings, and serve or store.

Boil

1. Place chicken in a large pot and add enough water to cover it completely.
2. Cover the pot and bring the water to a boil.
3. Reduce heat to a simmer and gently boil for 60 minutes.
4. Remove chicken, let cool, and shred or chop the meat.
5. Add seasonings, and serve or store.

Bake

1. Preheat oven to 400°F.
2. Spray baking sheet or dish with nonstick cooking spray, or line with foil or parchment paper.
3. Bake for 20–25 minutes or until chicken is no longer pink in the center and juices run clear.
4. Add seasonings, and serve or store.

Broil

1. Preheat oven to broil.
2. Spray broiler pan with nonstick cooking spray.
3. Butterfly-cut the chicken.
4. Move oven rack to the top.
5. Broil for 8 minutes per side.
6. Add seasonings, serve, or store.

Ground Turkey or Beef

Skillet or Frying Pan

1. Lightly spray large skillet or pan with nonstick cooking spray.
2. Cook the ground turkey or beef over medium heat for 5–10 minutes.
3. While cooking, continue to chop and break chicken into smaller and smaller chunks until browned.
4. Add seasonings, serve, or store.

Eggs

Hard-Boil

1. Bring a large pot of water to a boil.
2. Using a large spoon, carefully place each egg in the boiling water one at a time. Bring water back to a boil and let cook 10 minutes.
3. Drain and run cold water over the eggs until cool to touch.
4. Cool in fridge. Peel when ready to eat.

CARBS

Brown Rice

Cooked on the Stovetop

1. Place pot on the stove and add water and brown rice (for every 1 cup of brown rice, add 1½ cups water).
2. Bring water to a boil, cover with a lid, reduce heat, and simmer for 50 minutes.
3. Remove from heat and fluff with a fork.
4. Add seasonings, and serve or store.

Cooked in a Grain Cooker

1. Pour brown rice and water into the grain cooker (for every 1 cup brown rice, add 1½ cups water).
2. Close the lid and press START.
3. When cooked, open lid slowly and fluff with a fork.
4. Add seasonings, serve, or store.

Quinoa

Cooked on the Stovetop

1. Rinse quinoa with cold running water.
2. Follow directions on package.

Potatoes and Sweet Potatoes

Boil

1. Chop potatoes or yams and place in a pot.
2. Fill with water so that they are just covered.
3. Bring to a boil, reduce heat, and simmer for 50–60 minutes.
4. Remove from the heat and run under cold water until cool.
5. Add seasonings. Serve (with skins or mashed) or store.

Bake (chopped)

1. Preheat oven to 425°F.
2. Cover baking sheet with foil and spray with nonstick cooking spray.
3. Slice sweet potatoes into rounds or dice into cubes.
4. Bake 20 minutes. Flip. Bake another 15–20 minutes or until fork tender (not hard, but not mushy).

Bake (whole)

1. Preheat oven to 350°F.
2. Stab potatoes or yams with fork 8–10 times each to penetrate the skin.
3. Wrap each potato or yam in aluminum foil (optional).
4. Bake for 60 minutes.
5. Remove from oven and allow to cool for 30 minutes before serving or storing.

APPENDIX D

EXTREME CYCLE ACCEPTABLE FOODS AND 100-CALORIE PORTIONS

CARBS

Breads
Breads, whole-grain	1 slice
Tortillas, brown rice	¾ tortilla
Tortillas, corn	1½ tortillas

Cereal
All-Bran	½ cup
Fiber One	1 cup
Granola (low-fat)	⅓ cup
Kashi cereals	½ cup
Oatmeal	¾ cup

Fruits
Apples	1½ apple
Apricots	5 apricots
Bananas	1 banana
Berries	1½ cups
Grapes	1½ cups
Kiwi	3 kiwi
Lemon juice	8 ounces
Lime juice	8 ounces
Melons	2 cups
Monk fruit	Unlimited!
Oranges/Tangerines	1 whole
Peaches/Nectarines	2 whole
Pears	1 pear
Pineapple	1 cup
Plums	3 plums

Grains
Amaranth	½ cup
Barley	½ cup
Buckwheat	½ cup
Couscous	½ cup
Popcorn (air-popped)	3½ cups
Quinoa	½ cup
Rice, brown (long-grain)	½ cup
Rice, wild	½ cup

Legumes
Beans (low-sodium only)	½ cup
Hummus	2 tablespoons
Lentils (low-sodium only)	½ cup

Starchy Veggies
Carrots	2 cups
Corn	½ cup
Peas	1 cup
Potatoes (medium)	1 potato
Sweet potatoes/Yams (medium)	¾ cup

Pasta
Pasta, brown rice	½ cup
Pasta, whole-grain	½ cup

CONDIMENTS/DRESSINGS/MISC

Chili paste	½ tablespoon
Chili sauce	1½ tablespoons
Marinara sauce (Newman's Own)	½ cup
Mayonnaise (fat-free)	4 tablespoons
Mustard	6 teaspoons
Nonstick cooking spray (butter flavor)	10 sprays
Salad dressing, creamy	1.5 tablespoons
Salad dressing, French (fat-free)	4 tablespoons
Salad dressing, Italian (low-fat)	2 tablespoons
Salsa (Newman's Own All-Natural)	12 tablespoons
Soy sauce (low-sodium)	6 teaspoons
Tabasco sauce	20 teaspoons
Tomato paste	4 tablespoons
Tomato sauce	1 cup
Vinaigrette, balsamic (fat-free)	2 tablespoons
Vinegar, balsamic	2 tablespoons

EXTREME CYCLE ACCEPTABLE FOODS
AND 100-CALORIE PORTIONS

FATS

Almond butter (with salt)	1 tablespoon
Almond milk (unsweetened)	2 cups
Almonds (raw, whole)	2 tablespoons
Avocados	½ medium
Butter	1 tablespoon
Cheese	1 ounce
Cream, heavy whipping	2 tablespoons
Feta cheese/Ricotta cheese (regular)	⅓ cup
Mayonnaise (regular)	1 tablespoon
Oil, fish	1 tablespoon
Oil, flaxseed	1 tablespoon
Oil, olive	1 tablespoon
Olives (large)	10 olives
Peanut butter (powdered)	4.5 tablespoons
Peanut butter (salted)	1 tablespoon
Pecans (raw, chopped)	2 tablespoons
Sunflower seeds	2 tablespoons
Soy nuts (roasted, lightly salted)	2 tablespoons
Walnuts (raw, chopped)	2 tablespoons

HERBS & SPICES

Basil	Unlimited!
Cayenne pepper	Unlimited!
Chili powder	Unlimited!
Cinnamon	Unlimited!
Cloves	Unlimited!
Cocoa powder	Unlimited!
Curry powder	Unlimited!
Garlic/Garlic powder	Unlimited!
Ginger	Unlimited!
Horseradish	Unlimited!
Salt-free spice blends	Unlimited!
Nutmeg	Unlimited!
Onion powder	Unlimited!
Oregano	Unlimited!
Paprika	Unlimited!
Parsley	Unlimited!
Pepper, black	Unlimited!
Peppers	Unlimited!
Rosemary	Unlimited!
Sea salt (high-sodium)	Unlimited!
Stevia	Unlimited!
Thyme	Unlimited!
Turmeric	Unlimited!

PROTEIN

Egg substitutes	1 cup
Egg whites	5 whites
Egg yolks	2 yolks
Whey/Egg/Pea/ Soy protein powder	1 scoop

Beef

Steak, cube	2½ ounces
Steak, flank	2 ounces
Steak, round	2 ounces

Dairy

Cottage cheese	1 cup
Yogurt, fat-free plain Greek	1 cup

Lean Meats

Buffalo (ground)	1½ ounces
Chicken breast (lean ground)	2 ounces
Turkey (lean ground)	3 ounces
Ostrich/Duck breast	2 ounces
Venison/Elk	2 ounces

Poultry

Chicken breast	4 ounces
Chicken broth (low-sodium)	4 cups
Chicken thighs	3 ounces
Turkey breast (not deli)	3 ounces
Turkey (low-sodium deli)	3½ ounces

Seafood

Salmon (canned)	3½ ounces
Salmon (fillet)	2 ounces
Shellfish: Scallops/Crab/ Lobster/Shrimp	4 ounces
Tuna (canned)	3 ounces
Whitefish: Snapper/ Halibut/Cod/Tilapia	2 ounces

EXTREME CYCLE ACCEPTABLE FOODS
AND 100-CALORIE PORTIONS

VEGETABLES

Asparagus	Unlimited!
Broccoli	Unlimited!
Cabbage	Unlimited!
Cauliflower	Unlimited!
Celery	Unlimited!
Collard greens	Unlimited!
Cucumbers	Unlimited!
Eggplant	Unlimited!
Green beans	Unlimited!
Lettuces	Unlimited!
Mixed greens	Unlimited!
Mushrooms	Unlimited!
Onions	Unlimited!
Peppers	Unlimited!
Sprouts	Unlimited!
Squash	Unlimited!
Tomatoes	Unlimited!
Zucchini	Unlimited!

ACKNOWLEDGMENTS

A very special thank-you to the incredible team of stellar individuals who worked long and tireless hours to make this book possible: Billie Fitzpatrick, Simon Green, Ryan Levine, Jennifer Weaver, Molly Schoneveld, Hachette Books, Lisa LaFon, Erika Peterson, David Rushing, Allison Tyler Jones, Susan Kelley, and Jessie Dahling.

To our family and friends: Thank you for loving and supporting us unconditionally. Thank you for understanding our chaotic family life and work schedules. Even though we don't get to see much of one another these crazy days, we look forward to spending quality time together soon.

To ABC and our *Extreme Weight Loss* production crew: Thank you for your support, hard work, and friendship over the years. It has been a wild ride, but together we have been able to capture and share what the true journey of transformation looks like.

To our courageous *Extreme Weight Loss* participants: Thank you for letting us embark on the journey with you. Thank you for sharing your struggles and triumphs. Thank you for teaching us the real journey of transformation through your experiences. Because of you, we are able to share this guide with the world. Together, we will continue to change millions of lives.

INDEX

Want more inspiration and transformation?

Choose Chris Powell's other bestselling titles today!

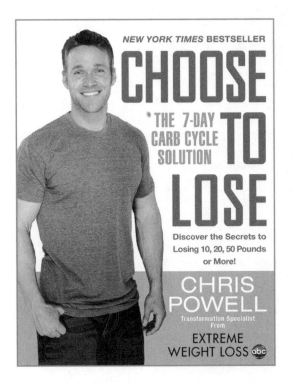

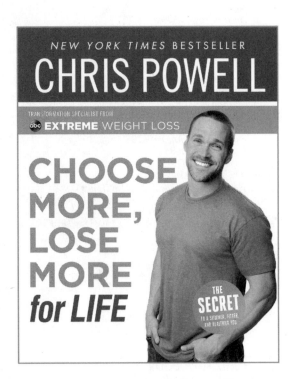

Also Available as eBooks and from
Hachette Audio

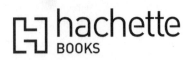